WALL PILA

FOR

WEIGHT LOSS

The Ultimate And Effective Workouts Routines For Maximum Weight Loss Suitable For Beginners, Seniors And Women Of All Ages With 28 Day Meal Plan To Keep You Fit

Ashley J. Nolen

BOOKS BY SAME AUTHOR

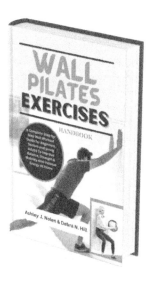

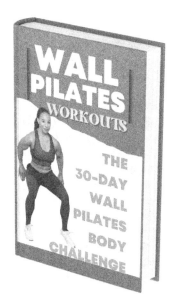

SCAN TO BUY

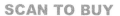

SCAN TO BUY

Copyright © Ashley J. Nolen, 2023.

Table of Contents

INTRODUCTION

As a seasoned practitioner of the distinctive and empowering exercise regimen known as wall Pilates, I have personally witnessed the remarkable and transformative effects it can have. Through the seamless integration of strength, flexibility, and mindfulness, wall Pilates has become a profound source of inspiration, propelling me on a journey of self-discovery, self-care, and holistic healing.

Embracing the wall as a stalwart ally, I have unlocked a realm of boundless possibilities in my fitness routine. The wall has become a sturdy pillar of support, empowering me to push beyond my perceived limitations, transcend my boundaries, and achieve extraordinary results. This journey has been nothing short of awe-inspiring, encompassing a newfound sense of body awareness, control, and alignment as I engage my core, elongate my spine, and flow through each exercise with an orchestrated symphony of grace and strength.

One of the most notable aspects of my personal voyage with wall Pilates has been its profound impact on my weight loss journey. As a dedicated fitness enthusiast, I have experimented with various exercise modalities, but wall Pilates has truly been a game-changer in my pursuit of a healthier, fitter self. The unique combination of resistance training, stretching, and breath work in wall Pilates has ignited my metabolism, sculpted my muscles, and accelerated my weight loss journey in ways I could have never imagined.

Yet, it's not solely about shedding pounds. Wall Pilates has instilled in me a deep sense of self-care and self-love, fostering a reverential relationship with my body. Through mindful movement and conscious breathing, I have cultivated a profound connection with my physical being, tapping into its inherent wisdom and unlocking its boundless potential.

The holistic approach of wall Pilates has transcended beyond the physical realm, profoundly impacting my mind and soul as well.

The practice has become a sanctuary, a haven where I can disconnect from the external chaos and tune into my inner being. The rhythmic flow of movement, the deep connection with my breath, and the meditative quality of wall Pilates have bestowed upon me a sense of peace, clarity, and mindfulness that resonates like never before.

As a seasoned wall Pilates instructor, I have witnessed the profound impact of this practice on my clients as well. From novices to advanced practitioners, I have witnessed lives transformed, bodies strengthened, and minds rejuvenated through the powerful effects of wall Pilates. It is a privilege to witness the joy, the sense of accomplishment, and the newfound confidence that my clients experience as they embark on their own personal journeys with this practice.

For those seeking to embark on their own transformational journey with wall Pilates, I wholeheartedly encourage you to take the leap and discover the inherent power of this practice for yourself. Whether you're a fitness enthusiast, a beginner, or someone looking to reignite your passion for movement, wall Pilates offers something truly extraordinary for everyone.

Understanding The Powerful Combination Of Wall Pilates And Weight Loss

New workout methods and approaches are continuously appearing in the fitness industry, promising to provide results that are unmatched. Wall Pilates, a distinctive and dynamic approach to exercise that combines the strength of Pilates with the use of a wall as a prop, is one such technique that has been gaining popularity in recent years. In my experience as a seasoned practitioner in the realm of Pilates training, wall Pilates' transforming benefits when included in a weight reduction programme have been seen personally. Let's go further into the nuances of wall Pilates in this thorough investigation and how it may be a powerful instrument for obtaining success in weight reduction endeavours.

Pilates is, at its heart, a complete method of exercise that goes beyond just physical fitness and incorporates components of strength, flexibility, balance, and body awareness. By use the wall as a prop, Wall Pilates elevates this kind of exercise by introducing a multiple degree of difficulty and support. The resistance and stability the wall offers via a sequence of exercises done on or with its assistance amplifies the workout's efficacy, making wall Pilates a force to be reckoned with in the world of fitness.

The fact that wall Pilates engages the core muscles in a distinctive and intense way is one of the main factors contributing to its effectiveness as a weight reduction strategy. The wall provides the body with a solid surface against which it may push, pull, and stabilise, profoundly engaging the abdominal, back, and pelvic muscles. Enhancing core stability, strength, and posture as a consequence of this strong core activation may be beneficial for both weight reduction and general physical fitness.

Wall Pilates is also a very versatile type of exercise that can be customised to meet individual goals and fitness levels, making it accessible to a wide variety of people, even those who may be beginners on their weight reduction journey. The utilisation of the wall as a prop offers a strong basis for adjustments and advancements, supporting a range of talents and objectives. With the capacity to be tailored to test and push one's limitations, regardless of their fitness level, wall Pilates is suited for both beginning and experienced practitioners.

Wall Pilates promotes flexibility and balance, two crucial elements of general fitness and weight reduction success, in addition to its core-strengthening advantages. Numerous wall Pilates exercises include the body being stretched, extended, and reaching in different directions, which improves flexibility and range of motion. As a consequence, you may perform better in sports, have higher muscle tone, and have better posture, all of which help you develop a more streamlined and toned figure as you lose weight.

As it tests the body's ability to retain stability and control while completing exercises on or with the help of the wall, the balance component of wall Pilates is equally important. This necessitates enhanced balance and coordination due to increased proprioception, or the body's sense of its location in space. Improved balance and coordination are not only essential for daily tasks but also work as a preventative measure against falls and accidents, particularly as one gets older.

Additionally, wall Pilates encourages mindfulness and body awareness, two things that may have a significant influence on efforts to lose weight. One must be totally present in the moment, deliberately engage the muscles, and pay attention to the breath when doing wall Pilates movements. This attention may penetrate other facets of life, including eating behaviours, in addition to the exercise session. It makes it easier to limit portion sizes and make appropriate meal selections since it helps one become more sensitive to the body's signals of hunger and fullness.

In addition to its physical advantages, wall Pilates is good for one's mental and emotional health, which may significantly aid weight reduction attempts. Regular wall Pilates practise may help lower stress, elevate mood, boost confidence, and improve perception of one's physique. Through wall Pilates, you may increase your strength, flexibility, and balance as well as your feeling of control over your own body. These benefits can help you be more motivated and dedicated to your weight reduction quest.

Additionally, wall Pilates encourages you to listen to your body's messages, acknowledge its limits, and work with it rather than against it in order to foster a healthy mind-body connection. By using a mindful approach to exercise, you may create a better connection with your body and get a greater understanding of both its potential and its limits. As you learn to place a higher priority on self-care and self-compassion, this may result in a more joyful and long-lasting approach to weight reduction.

Pilates on a wall may be included into your weight reduction programme to provide diversity and enjoyment. Your exercises will be more challenging and creative by using the wall as a prop, which will make them more fun and interesting. You may choose from a variety of exercises at Wall Pilates that can be tailored to meet your interests and fitness objectives so that you can continue to push yourself and improve over time. Due to the diversity, you'll look forward to your wall Pilates sessions and enjoy the process of discovering new moves and sensations, which will help you remain motivated and devoted to your weight reduction objectives.

For the best weight reduction outcomes, wall Pilates should be used with a good, balanced diet, just like any other workout programme. While doing wall Pilates may increase your strength, flexibility, and body awareness, it's equally vital to focus on your diet and other lifestyle choices. A comprehensive strategy that incorporates wall Pilates with a good eating plan, enough sleep, and stress reduction strategies may provide a synergistic impact that supports your weight loss objectives and aids in the achievement of long-lasting results.

How This Book Will Help You Achieve Your Weight Loss Goals with Wall Pilates

The book "Achieving Weight Loss Goals with Wall Pilates" is a comprehensive guide that provides you with a step-by-step plan to incorporate wall pilates into your fitness routine and achieve your weight loss goals. Here's how this book can help you:

Detailed Instructions: The book provides detailed instructions on how to perform wall pilates exercises correctly and safely, with clear explanations and illustrations. It includes guidance on proper form, breathing techniques, and modifications for different fitness levels, ensuring that you can perform the exercises effectively.

Structured Workout Plans: The book offers structured workout plans that are specifically designed for weight loss. These plans include a variety of wall pilates exercises that target different muscle groups and provide a well-rounded workout. The plans also outline recommended sets, repetitions, and duration for each exercise, making it easy for you to follow along and track your progress.

Focus on Wall Pilates for Weight Loss: Unlike traditional pilates, which is typically done on a mat, this book focuses on wall pilates as a unique approach for weight loss. Wall pilates incorporates the use of a wall for support, which adds resistance and challenge to the exercises, helping you build strength, flexibility, and endurance. The book explains how wall pilates can help you burn calories, tone your muscles, and improve your overall fitness level, making it an effective tool for weight loss.

Comprehensive Information: The book provides comprehensive information on the benefits of wall pilates for weight loss, including how it can help you improve your posture, increase your muscle tone, and enhance your mind-body connection. It also discusses the importance of proper nutrition and hydration for weight loss, and how to incorporate these principles into your lifestyle to optimize your results.

Practical Tips and Strategies: The book includes practical tips and strategies to help you stay motivated, overcome challenges, and sustain your weight loss goals. It provides guidance on setting realistic goals, creating a routine, and staying consistent with your wall pilates practice. It also offers suggestions on how to make healthy choices in your diet and lifestyle, and how to maintain a positive mindset throughout your weight loss journey.

CHAPTER ONE

What is wall Pilates?

Wall Pilates is a unique form of exercise that combines Pilates techniques with the use of a wall for support and resistance. It involves performing Pilates exercises while utilizing the wall as a prop for stability, alignment, and additional challenge. Wall Pilates can be done using a variety of equipment such as resistance bands, exercise balls, and small props like hand weights or foam rollers, along with the support of the wall.

It focuses on core strengthening, flexibility, balance, and body awareness. The wall provides support and stability, allowing practitioners to better engage their core muscles and maintain proper alignment throughout the exercises. It also offers resistance, which adds an extra challenge to the movements and helps to build strength and tone muscles.

Benefits of WALL Pilates

Enhancing Core Strength

Strengthening the core muscles, which comprise the pelvic floor muscles, back muscles, and abdominal muscles, is one of the fundamental tenets of Pilates. WALL Pilates goes one step further by use the wall as a prop, adding extra support and resistance to even more fully work the core muscles. Improved core strength may be attained via regular Wall Pilates practise, which is necessary for maintaining stability, balance, and correct alignment during exercise and everyday activities.

Increased Flexibility

Another vital component of fitness that Pilates emphasises is flexibility. Stretching activities are a part of WALL Pilates, which serve to increase the flexibility of the muscles and joints. Stretching may be done safely and effectively with the assistance of the wall, which can aid in injury prevention and increase general flexibility. By enabling a broader range of motion during exercise and resulting in more effective workouts and improved calorie burn, increased flexibility may also help with weight reduction.

Improved Posture

In addition to being significant for appearance, good posture is also crucial for general health and wellbeing. Muscle imbalances, back discomfort, and decreased functional capacity may all be caused by poor posture. WALL Pilates emphasises good spinal alignment and pushes postural muscle activation to create better posture. By using the wall as a prop, you may get support and feedback, which will help you align your spine and activate your postural muscles, which will gradually improve your posture.

Stress Relief

Today's fast-paced society has made stress a prevalent component of many people's lives. By raising cortisol levels, which may cause hormonal imbalances and comfort food cravings, high levels of stress can have a detrimental influence on weight reduction attempts. Breathing exercises and deliberate movements used in WALL Pilates may help lower stress and encourage relaxation. A more balanced and concentrated approach to weight reduction is possible with the emphasis on deep breathing and mindful exercise, which may help relax the mind and relieve stress.

How WALL Pilates Supports Weight Loss

We now have a solid knowledge of WALL Pilates and its broad advantages, so let's explore how WALL Pilates promotes weight reduction particularly.

Engages the Core Muscles

WALL Pilates has a strong emphasis on activating the core, as was already discussed. When used as a prop, the wall offers support and resistance, enabling focused activation of the core muscles during workouts. In addition to helping tonify and develop the abdominal muscles, using the core muscles also encourages improved posture and stability. A strong core is necessary for appropriate body alignment and effective movement, which may reduce the risk of accidents and enhance weight-loss activities.

Promotes Muscle Toning

WALL Pilates focuses the arms, legs, glutes, and back in addition to the key muscular areas in the core. A resistance training exercise that uses regulated motions and the resistance of a wall may help tone and shape muscles. Muscles that are toned not only seem more defined, but they also burn more calories when at rest, which may help people lose weight. By using WALL Pilates to develop lean muscle mass, you may boost your metabolism generally and burn calories more effectively, even when you're not doing out.

Enhances Metabolism

Weight reduction depends heavily on metabolism. An increased metabolism causes the body to burn more calories when at rest, which may aid in weight reduction. With its emphasis on muscular activation and tone, WALL Pilates may assist increase metabolism.

As was previously noted, lean muscle mass is increased by resistance exercise, and toned muscles burn more calories when at rest. Additionally, the WALL Pilates' deep breathing and mindful movement methods may enhance the blood flow to and oxygenation of the muscles, promoting metabolism and calorie burning even more.

Enhances Cardiovascular Health

In order to lose weight and maintain overall fitness, cardiovascular health is crucial. Exercises that boost heart rate and enhance endurance include cycling, jogging, and brisk walking. Although WALL Pilates is not seen as a typical cardiovascular workout, it may nevertheless have positive effects for the heart. When coupled with continuous, fluid motions, using the wall as resistance produces a demanding exercise that raises heart rate. WALL Pilates may promote weight reduction attempts and enhance cardiovascular health since it increases heart rate and improves circulation.

Encourages Mindful Eating

Exercise alone won't help you lose weight; you also need to adopt appropriate eating practises. The emphasis on mindfulness in WALL Pilates is one of its distinctive features. The WALL Pilates techniques of deep breathing, focus, and mind-body connection may be used outside of the gym to daily life, including food practises. The principles of mindful eating include eating with purpose and without interruption while being completely present and aware of the eating experience. By improving awareness of hunger and fullness signals, lowering emotional eating, and boosting mindful food choices, the mindfulness component of Wall Pilates may help good eating practises.

Tips for Incorporating WALL Pilates into Your Weight Loss Routine

Now that you are aware of how WALL Pilates can support weight loss, here are some tips for incorporating WALL Pilates into your weight loss routine:

Start with a Qualified Instructor or Instruction Manuals: It is advised to start with a Qualified Instructor or Instruction Manuals if you are new to WALL Pilates or exercise in general. Depending on your fitness level and objectives, a qualified Pilates teacher or instruction manuals may provide advice on appropriate form, technique, and adaptations. This guarantees that you are exercising safely and properly, maximising the weight-loss advantages of WALL Pilates.

The Key Is Consistency The key to any exercise regimen is consistency. For the greatest benefits, aim for consistent WALL Pilates sessions, preferably twice weekly. Make WALL Pilates a regular part of your weight reduction programme and commit to a schedule.

Increasing the intensity and complexity of the exercises progressively can help you become more comfortable with WALL Pilates. This may be accomplished by increasing the amount of resistance, the number of repetitions, or by moving on to harder exercises. Gradual progression encourages ongoing development by presenting your muscles with new challenges.

WALL Pilates has many advantages for weight reduction, but it's crucial to combine it with cardiovascular workouts like fast walking, jogging, or cycling to maximise calorie burn and improve fitness in general. A healthy, balanced diet must also be followed in order to successfully lose weight. To assist your weight reduction objectives, include full, nutrient-dense meals in your diet and pay attention to portion sizes.

During WALL Pilates workouts, pay close attention to your body and pay heed to its suggestions. If you experience any discomfort or pain, stop the exercise and alter it, or ask your teacher for advice. As pushing yourself too far might result in injury or setbacks in your weight reduction efforts, it's important to respect your body's limitations.

Setting up Your Wall Pilates Workout Space for Success

Having a dedicated space that is specially set up for your exercises may have a significant influence on your performance and growth while doing Pilates. Utilising the wall is one practical method to design a room that is ideal for Pilates workouts.

How therefore can you optimise your wall Pilates exercise area? Let's start now!

Locate the proper location: Finding the ideal location is the first step in building up your wall Pilates exercise area. The ideal location in your house is one that is roomy, well-ventilated, and has a flat, unobstructed wall. Ensure that there is sufficient room for you to walk about comfortably and that there are no obstructions or distractions on the wall. You may concentrate and devote yourself totally to your Pilates practise in a clutter-free and calm setting.

assemble the essential tools: Getting the tools you'll need for your wall Pilates exercise is the next step. To provide your body support and grip, you'll need a sticky mat or a yoga mat. For certain exercises, you'll also need a small towel or folded blanket to support your head and neck. A resistance band or strap is also necessary to increase the difficulty of your activities. You'll be able to go through your Pilates exercise without pauses if you have these fundamental props available and ready to use.

Establish a visual focal point: During your Pilates practise, a visual focal point may be a useful tool for helping you remain motivated and concentrated. To assist you in maintaining perfect alignment and form, think about adding a focus point to the wall in front of you. This might be a straightforward poster, a work of art, or even a motivating saying that speaks to you. Your training area may benefit from having a visual focal point by adding a touch of aesthetics and making it more appealing and motivating.

Keep it useful and organised: It's essential for your success to keep your wall Pilates training area functional and organised. Ensure that all of your equipment, including your mat, towel, resistance band, and strap, is put neatly and is simple to use. To keep your props neat and organised, utilise shelves, hooks, or storage bins. Additionally, ensure sure your wall anchors are firmly fastened and that the resistance band or strap you're using for your workouts is set correctly. Your Pilates exercise will go more quickly and easily if your training area is organised and practical.

Establish a peaceful setting since it has a big influence on your Pilates practise. You may unwind, concentrate, and completely participate in your exercises by setting a relaxing mood in your wall Pilates training area. Think about including calming aspects like soft lighting, peaceful colours, and relaxing music. To create a calm atmosphere, you may also include organic components like plants or diffusers of essential oils. Your whole experience might be improved by a tranquil setting, which enables you to completely connect with your body and mind throughout your Pilates practise.

Personalise your training area: By making your wall Pilates practise area special to you, you may increase the fun and motivation of your sessions. Think of including unique elements that express your sense of fashion, taste, and individuality. It may be pieces of art, inspirational sayings, or sentimental objects that have unique importance to you. You'll be more inclined to utilise your area often and consistently if you personalise it since it will give you a feeling of ownership and pride.

Take safety measures into account: Setting up your wall Pilates training area should always put safety first. Make that your wall anchors are properly installed, can sustain the weight of your body, and can accommodate a resistance band or strap. To avoid injuries, do your workouts with good form and alignment. Consult a certified Pilates teacher or other fitness expert for advice if you have questions about a certain exercise or technique. You may practise Pilates in your wall exercise area securely and productively by taking the required safety measures.

Wall Pilates Equipments

Using a wall while doing Pilates exercises may significantly improve your workout. A wall may provide resistance, stability, and support, enabling you to carry out a variety of workouts that focus on different muscle areas. Additionally, include a wall in your Pilates programme might help you lose weight by making your routines more challenging and intense. But you'll need the appropriate equipment to create a good and productive wall Pilates practise. In order to set up your training area for success, we'll look at the necessary equipment for wall Pilates and weight reduction in this post.

Why Use Equipment for Wall Pilates?

You may concentrate on your form, alignment, and use of the appropriate muscles by using the wall to offer stability and support. The wall may also increase resistance, making your workouts harder and more effective at increasing strength and flexibility. Utilising equipment made expressly for wall Pilates may increase the advantages of this exercise even further.

Essential Wall Pilates Equipment

Consider these necessary pieces of equipment for your wall Pilates practise:

A wall-mounted bar is a reliable and adaptable piece of equipment that can be fastened to the wall at different heights. For workouts like leg circles, pull-ups, and other hanging activities, it offers stability and support. Look for a bar that is firmly fastened to the wall and constructed of sturdy materials.

restraining bands Elastic bands known as resistance bands may be fastened to a wall to provide resistance to your workouts. They let you to alter the intensity of your exercise since they have different degrees of resistance. Exercises like arm, leg, and core training may all be done using resistance bands.

Pilates/Yoga Mat: When doing floor workouts, a supportive, non-slip mat is crucial for cushioning and supporting your body. To avoid slipping and sliding while working out, look for a mat that is thick enough to provide appropriate cushioning and has a non-slip surface.

Pilates Ball: You may do a number of exercises with a Pilates ball, sometimes referred to as a stability ball or exercise ball, to test your stability and core strength. It may be positioned between you and the wall to make exercises like squats, bridges, and sitting twists more difficult.

Dumbbells, commonly referred to as hand weights, may be used to provide resistance to arm workouts, enhancing their capacity to develop upper body strength. Make sure the weights you choose are suitable for your level of fitness and your objectives, and keep them safely when not in use.

Ankle Weights: You may increase resistance to lower body movements like leg lifts, hamstring curls, and inner thigh pushes by wearing ankle weights around your ankles. Choose ankle weights that are stable and pleasant to wear so that they won't shift about while you work out.

Exercise Ring: A flexible circular-shaped ring, commonly referred to as a magic circle or a Pilates ring, may be used for support and resistance during a variety of activities. It may be positioned between you and the wall to intensify your Pilates workout and test your muscles.

Mirror: When doing wall Pilates, a mirror may be a useful aid for checking your form and alignment. It enables you to determine if you are carrying out the exercises properly and may help you make modifications to enhance your technique.

How to Choose the Right Equipment

There are a few crucial things to think about while choosing equipment for your wall Pilates practise:

Quality and Durability: Select equipment that is constructed from top-notch components and is built to survive repeated usage. Equipment that is built to endure a long time and provide dependable support and resistance throughout your exercises is something you should invest in.

Equipment that is readily adjusted to your height, degree of fitness, and preferred exercises should be used. You may execute a greater variety of workouts using equipment that is adjustable, and it can be customised to meet your unique demands.

When choosing equipment for your wall Pilates practise, comfort is crucial. Look for equipment with features like padded handles, non-slip surfaces, and ergonomic designs to make it more pleasant to use. Your exercises will be more pleasurable and productive if you have comfortable equipment.

Safety: When choosing equipment for any kind of activity, safety should come first. Make that the apparatus is stable, firmly fastens to the wall, and has the necessary safety features, such as non-slip surfaces and strong fastenings. In order to avoid injuries, it's crucial to use the equipment as directed and adhere to good form and technique.

Consider using equipment that is versatile and can be utilised for a variety of activities. This enables you to change up your exercises and focus on other muscle areas, enhancing the versatility and efficacy of your wall Pilates routine.

CHAPTER TWO

The Science Behind Weight Loss And Pilates

Diet, exercise, and lifestyle choices are just a few of the many elements that go into the complicated process of losing weight. Pilates, which places an emphasis on power, flexibility, and core stability, may help with weight reduction when paired with other healthy lifestyle modifications.

Calorie Balance: A key idea in weight management, calorie balance describes the harmony between the calories you intake and the calories you expend via physical activity and metabolism. It is very important in deciding whether you put on weight, lose weight, or keep it off. It's crucial to comprehend and control calorie balance if you want to lose weight in a healthy and long-lasting way.

Simply defined, weight loss happens when you generate a calorie deficit, or when you expend more calories than you take in. On the other hand, weight gain happens when you ingest a calorie surplus—more calories than you burn. When you have a calorie balance—that is, when you take in and expend the same quantity of calories—you will stay at your present weight. You can efficiently regulate your body weight by controlling your calorie balance.

Let's explore the idea of calorie balance in more detail and see how it affects your efforts to lose weight:

Calorie Intake: Your calorie intake, or the quantity of calories you take in through food and drinks, is the primary factor in calorie balancing. When you eat, your body digests the food and releases calories as fuel for various bodily activities including metabolism, exercise, and other physiological processes. Your calorie intake is significantly influenced by the kind and quantity of food you eat.

It's critical to consume less calories than your body requires for normal functioning if you want to lose weight. A balanced, nutritious diet high in whole foods like fruits, vegetables, lean proteins, healthy fats, and complex carbs will help you accomplish this. Compared to processed meals, sugary drinks, and high-fat snacks, these nutrient-dense foods provide vital vitamins, minerals, and other nutrients while having less calories.

Controlling your portions is essential for controlling your calorie consumption. You may prevent ingesting too many calories that might cause weight gain by being aware of serving sizes and avoiding large quantities. Making healthy meal choices may be aided by keeping track of your calorie consumption using tools like food diaries or calorie monitoring apps.

Calorie Expenditure: Your calorie expenditure, or the quantity of calories you burn via physical activity, exercise, and metabolism, is the second factor in calorie balance. Any movement you do during the day, such as walking, jogging, cycling, swimming, and other types of exercise, is considered physical activity. The term "exercise" on the other hand describes physical activity that is organised and planned with the intention of enhancing fitness and wellbeing.

Exercise and physical activity both help you burn more calories, which may help you achieve a calorie deficit and lose weight. Exercises that increase cardiovascular fitness, such as running, cycling, or brisk walking, are good at burning calories. Exercises for building muscle mass, like weightlifting or resistance training, may also help you burn more calories even while you're at rest since they speed up your metabolism.

Your metabolism, in addition to physical activity and exercise, affects how many calories you burn. The quantity of calories your body requires to sustain fundamental physiological processes including breathing, digesting, and circulation when at rest is referred to as basal metabolic rate (BMR). Your BMR may be affected by factors including age, gender, body composition, and genetics. For instance, having greater muscle mass might raise your BMR since it takes more energy to sustain muscles than fat does.

Making a Calorie Shortfall

You must expend more calories than you consume in order to produce a calorie deficit and lose weight. You may do this by controlling your calorie intake as well as your calorie expenditure. For instance, increasing your calorie expenditure via regular physical activity and exercise while decreasing your calorie intake through healthy food and portion management might result in a calorie deficit and support weight reduction.

The size of the calorie deficit necessary to lose weight is influenced by a number of variables, including your present weight, age, gender, level of exercise, and weight reduction objectives. A calorie deficit of 500 to 1000 calories per day is often advised for healthy and long-lasting weight reduction. As a consequence, you may lose 1 to 2 pounds every week, which is thought to be a safe and doable pace.

It's vital to remember that very calorie-restrictive diets or generating excessive calorie deficits might backfire, increase health risks, and cause muscle loss rather than fat reduction. Prioritising a healthy and long-term weight reduction strategy by establishing a manageable and lasting moderate calorie deficit is essential.

It might be beneficial to manage your calorie balance to measure and monitor your calorie intake and expenditure. In order to achieve a healthy calorie deficit for weight reduction, it might be helpful to keep a meal diary, use a calorie monitoring app, or speak with a licenced dietitian or nutritionist.

Nutrient Density: While controlling calorie balance is essential for weight reduction, it's also critical to take into account the nutrient density of the meals you eat. The term "nutrient density" describes the ratio of a food's quantity of calories to its amount of vital nutrients, such as vitamins, minerals, and antioxidants. Keeping your calorie consumption in control while eating nutrient-dense meals may help ensure that your body obtains the nutrients it needs for optimum health.

When opposed to processed and sugary meals, choosing whole, minimally processed foods like fruits, vegetables, lean meats, whole grains, and healthy fats may provide vital nutrients while being lower in calories. During your weight loss journey, eating foods high in nutrients may help you feel fuller for longer, maintain energy levels, and promote overall wellbeing.

Macronutrient balancing

For optimum weight reduction, it's crucial to balance the macronutrients in your diet in addition to taking your daily caloric intake into account. Carbohydrates, proteins, and fats are the three main nutrients that provide the body energy and are referred to as macronutrients. Optimising your weight reduction attempts may require balancing your consumption of these macronutrients.

Your diet should include carbs since they are the body's main energy source. However, it's vital to pick complex carbohydrates over refined ones like white bread, sugary meals, and drinks. Examples of such foods include whole grains, legumes, and vegetables. Proteins are necessary for the synthesis and repair of tissues. They also make you feel fuller for longer, which might help you lose weight. You may include lean protein sources in your diet, including tofu, fish, chicken, and beans. Healthy fats may also make you feel full and promote general health. Examples of these fats include those in nuts, seeds, avocados, and olive oil.

You may manage your calorie balance for weight reduction while maintaining a well-rounded and balanced diet by balancing the consumption of carbs, proteins, and fats.

Regular Physical Activity: As was already said, exercise and physical activity are essential for calorie burning and weight reduction. Regular exercise may help you lose weight, build muscle, speed up your metabolism, and feel better overall.

A well-rounded approach to physical activity may be achieved by including both cardiovascular exercises—such as walking, jogging, or swimming—and strength training—such as weightlifting or resistance training—into your programme. Aim for two or more days per week of strength training exercises that target the main muscle groups, coupled with at least 150 minutes per week of moderate-intensity aerobic activity, such as brisk walking or cycling.

The practise of mindful eating may significantly contribute to attaining a good calorie balance in addition to controlling calorie intake and expenditure. Paying attention to your body's hunger and fullness signals, eating deliberately, and savouring each meal while avoiding distractions like TV or cellphones are all parts of mindful eating. It also entails being conscious of your feelings and ideas towards food and eating.

By engaging in mindful eating, you may reduce overeating, encourage thoughtful meal selection, and establish a positive connection with food. Additionally, it may assist you in being more aware of your body's signals of hunger and fullness and help you stop mindless snacking and emotional eating, both of which can result in an unhealthily imbalanced calorie intake.

Sleep and Stress Management: Managing your stress and sleep patterns may have a significant impact on your calorie intake and weight reduction goals. Your hormonal balance, particularly the hormones that control appetite and fullness, such as leptin and ghrelin, may be upset by sleep deprivation or poor sleep quality. This may result in an increase in hunger and desires for foods that are rich in calories, which may result in an unfavourable calorie balance.

Similar to emotional eating, overeating, and poor food choices, excessive levels of stress may affect your calorie balance. To promote a healthy calorie balance and general well-being, it's critical to prioritise getting enough sleep and using stress management strategies like mindfulness, meditation, exercise, and relaxation methods.

Last but not least, maintaining a good calorie balance requires a long-term lifestyle modification rather than a one-time effort. Instead of relying on fast cures or fad diets, it's critical to approach weight reduction and calorie balancing with an emphasis on long-term sustainability. In order to lose weight in a sustainable manner, one must be consistent, patient, and committed.

A good calorie balance and long-term weight control may be achieved by making incremental, sustainable adjustments to your lifestyle, including how you eat, how much you exercise, and your general level of activity. Avoid excessive diets, severe calorie restrictions, and unsustainable workout routines that might harm your metabolism, muscle mass, and general health. Instead, concentrate on developing a balanced, healthy lifestyle that you can keep up over time.

A Healthful Diet

Maintaining a balanced diet and promoting overall wellbeing both depend on healthy eating. It entails making informed decisions about the foods you eat, taking their nutritional content and serving sizes into account. With a focus on full, nutrient-dense meals, a healthy eating plan often consists of a range of foods from all food categories in suitable amounts. Here are some essential guidelines for a healthy diet:

Balanced macronutrients are the three primary nutrient groups that provide the body energy: carbs, proteins, and fats. A healthy diet has a balance of these macronutrients. Since complex carbs like whole grains, fruits, and vegetables are the main source of energy, a healthy eating plan restricts simple carbohydrates like refined sugars and processed meals.

Lean meats, poultry, fish, eggs, legumes, nuts, and dairy products are good sources of protein, which is necessary for the growth and repair of tissues. Healthy fats, which are necessary for brain function and general health and should be ingested in moderation, include those in nuts, seeds, avocados, fatty fish, and olive oil.

Adequate Fibre Intake: Fibre is a form of carbohydrate that the body does not digest but instead travels through the digestive system mostly undigested. It has several health advantages, including aiding weight management, enhancing digestive health, and controlling blood sugar levels. Adequate fibre is part of a balanced diet and may be found in whole grains, fruits, vegetables, legumes, nuts, and seeds.

Foods that are abundant in vital nutrients, such as vitamins, minerals, and antioxidants, compared to their calorie content are referred to as nutrient-dense foods. Due to their ability to promote healthy biological processes and avoid nutritional shortages, these foods are crucial for general health and wellbeing. Colourful fruits and vegetables, lean proteins, whole grains, dairy products or dairy substitutes, and healthy fats are a few examples of foods that are nutrient-dense.

Portion Control: Keeping a healthy eating plan consistent requires paying close attention to portion proportions. Even nutritious meals might cause weight gain if they are taken in excess. It's crucial to pay attention to portion sizes as well as your body's signals of hunger and fullness. You may efficiently control portion sizes by avoiding eating directly from the container, using smaller plates, bowls and utensils, and doing so.

Limiting added sugars and salt: Eating too much added sugar and sodium may cause weight gain, high blood sugar, and high blood pressure, among other health problems. Limiting the intake of foods and drinks that are rich in added sugars, such as sugary drinks, desserts, and snacks, is a key component of a healthy eating plan. Additionally, it's crucial to choose lower-sodium options wherever feasible and restrict the consumption of high-sodium items such processed foods, canned foods, and restaurant meals.

A healthy eating plan places a strong emphasis on diversity and moderation. Eating a variety of meals from various food categories makes it easier to ensure that you get a variety of nutrients for optimum health. Additionally, moderation is essential since an imbalanced diet may result from consuming too much of any one food or vitamin. Aim for a well-rounded, balanced diet that includes a range of foods in reasonable amounts.

Avoiding Fad Diets: Although they sometimes promise immediate weight reduction, fad diets are neither sustainable nor healthful over the long run. They could discourage the eating of certain food categories, encourage severe caloric deficits, or stimulate the overconsumption of particular nutrients. Instead of relying on passing trends, a healthy eating plan emphasises sustainability, moderation, and a balanced diet.

Seeking Professional Advice: It's vital to obtain professional advice from a qualified dietitian or healthcare practitioner if you have particular dietary demands, medical issues, or weight reduction objectives. They are able to build a healthy eating plan that is customised to your particular demands based on your own needs, tastes, and health state.

Rest and restoration

Every workout regimen needs time for rest and recuperation. To avoid overtraining and lower the chance of injury, give your body enough time to recuperate in between sessions. Pay attention to your body's cues for relaxation and recuperation, get adequate sleep, and remain hydrated.

Before beginning any workout programme, it's crucial to speak with a healthcare professional, particularly if you have any underlying health disorders or worries. They can advise you on the forms and volumes of exercise that are secure and suitable for your particular need.

Personal Changes

An essential part of a successful weight reduction journey is making lifestyle modifications. It's important to develop long-lasting healthy habits rather than merely short-term diets and exercise routines. Changes in your way of life may assist you in achieving and maintaining a healthy weight, enhancing your general wellbeing, and preventing weight gain.

Here are three significant lifestyle adjustments that might aid your attempts to lose weight:

Meal preparation: Making healthy decisions and preventing impulsive eating are made possible with meal preparation. Make a grocery list, plan your meals and snacks, and go shopping for fresh vegetables, lean meats, and other nutritious products. As much as you can, prepare meals at home to have more control over the contents and serving sizes.

Physical activity: Losing weight and maintaining weight need regular exercise. Aim for 150 minutes or more per week of moderate-intensity aerobic exercise, such as brisk walking or cycling. Increase your metabolism by including strength training workouts to help you maintain and grow your muscle mass.

Sleep: Getting enough sleep is crucial for both weight reduction and general wellness. Hormones that control hunger and fullness may be disturbed by a lack of sleep, which can increase appetite and cause desires for unhealthy foods. To help your attempts to lose weight, aim for 7-9 hours of good sleep each night.

Stress reduction: Prolonged stress may cause emotional eating and impede weight loss. Use relaxation methods to reduce your stress levels, such as yoga, meditation, or deep breathing. Discover healthy coping mechanisms for stress, such as chatting to a friend, taking a stroll, or taking up a hobby.

Support network: Surrounding oneself with a strong network of friends and family may keep you inspired and responsible. Consult with friends, relatives, or a support group for assistance. To gain specialised advice and assistance, think about working with a licenced nutritionist, personal trainer, or healthcare provider.

Remind yourself that lifestyle changes need time and work, and practise patience with yourself. Significant weight reduction and an improvement in general health might result from gradual, small, sustained improvements. Celebrate your success along the road as you work to establish long-lasting healthy habits.

Mentality and Action

Achieving and sustaining weight reduction goals depends heavily on having the proper attitude and behaviour. It's important to address the psychological and behavioural aspects of weight control in addition to the physical ones. You may overcome obstacles, control emotional eating, establish long-term success, and create a healthy relationship with food by adopting a positive mentality and changing your behaviour.

Here are some significant mental and behavioural factors that might aid your attempts to lose weight:

By paying attention to your eating habits, being conscious of your hunger and fullness signals, and eating mindfully, you may create a better connection with food. Focus on the flavour, texture, and pleasure of your meals instead of being distracted by TV or other displays while you eat. You may improve digestion and prevent overeating by practising mindful eating.

Emotional eating: A lot of individuals use food as a coping mechanism for negative feelings like stress, grief, or boredom. You may control emotional eating by being aware of your emotional triggers and learning alternate coping mechanisms like exercise, meditation, or talking to a friend. You may be able to make better eating decisions if you can distinguish between actual and emotional hunger.

Self-Reflection and Self-Care: Taking the time to consider your ideas, feelings, and actions in relation to eating and losing weight may help you see trends and make the necessary adjustments. On your weight-loss journey, practise self-compassion, self-care, and kindness towards yourself. Celebrate your victories, take lessons from your failures, and concentrate on improvement rather than perfection.

Setting objectives: Setting goals that are attainable, quantifiable, and practical may keep you motivated and committed to your weight reduction journey. Your objectives should be broken down into smaller, more attainable stages. Regularly assess your progress. Celebrate your progress along the way and adjust your objectives as necessary. Clear objectives may give you a feeling of direction and purpose and can also help you stick with your weight reduction strategy.

Accountability: Being responsible for your actions and receiving support from others may both significantly improve your attempts to lose weight. Describe your objectives and progress to a close friend, member of your family, or a support group. To gain expert advice and assistance, think about working with a certified nutritionist, personal trainer, or therapist. You can keep motivated and on track by regularly checking in with people and getting their input.

Overcoming Obstacles: It's important to recognise and remove obstacles that can impede your weight reduction success. Lack of time, stress, awkward social settings, and cravings are common obstacles. Create plans for your meals, set aside time for exercise, identify healthy ways to deal with stress, or devise ways to handle social situations while maintaining an awareness of your food choices as ways to get around these obstacles.

Flexibility and Resilience: Losing weight is a process filled with ups and downs, therefore it's critical to have these qualities. Be willing to change your strategy as necessary, and be kind with yourself if you make a mistake. Learn from failures and take use of the chance to grow and make wiser decisions in the future. You may overcome obstacles and maintain your commitment to your weight reduction objectives by developing resilience and a positive outlook.

Tracking and Monitoring

A successful weight reduction journey requires constant monitoring and recording of your progress. You may get important insights, remain responsible, and make required changes to your plan by keeping track of what you eat, how much you exercise, and other pertinent data. Here are some pointers for efficient tracking and monitoring:

Food journaling: By keeping a food diary, you may better understand your eating patterns and make more informed decisions. Record everything you consume, including serving amounts and any snacks or sweets, in writing. Track your consumption frequently and enter information honestly. You may track your food consumption using a physical diary, a smartphone app, or an internet tool.

Regular Weigh-Ins: Keeping track of your weight will help you remain accountable and provide you feedback on your progress. Pick a regular day and time to weigh yourself, and note the information in a diary or tracking app. Focus on trends over time rather than daily swings since weight might change owing to a variety of variables, such as water retention or muscle building.

Monitoring your feelings, thoughts, and actions in relation to what you eat and how much you exercise may help you see triggers, trends, and opportunities for development. To keep note of your emotional state, stress levels, reasons why you eat emotionally, and any instances of thoughtless or impulsive eating, keep a diary or use a monitoring app. This might assist you in being more conscious of your actions and implementing healthy adjustments.

Hydration

A vital component of both weight reduction and general wellness is hydration. Numerous biological processes depend on maintaining sufficient hydration, which may also have a positive or negative influence on your efforts to lose weight. Here are some reasons why being well hydrated is important, as well as advice for doing so:

Water is calorie-free and may make you feel full and content, which can help you resist the need to snack on foods or beverages with lots of calories. You may assist your weight reduction goals by consuming fewer calories overall by drinking water before to or during meals.

Increases Metabolism: Your metabolism, which is the mechanism through which your body burns calories to create energy, may be supported by being hydrated. Dehydration may decrease your metabolism, making it more difficult for your body to burn calories effectively and perhaps preventing you from losing weight.

Energy and Performance: For optimum physical and mental performance, proper hydration is crucial. Being well hydrated increases your likelihood of having the strength and energy to do the regular exercise and physical activity that is essential for weight reduction.

Dehydration may cause weariness, cramping in the muscles, and impaired exercise performance, making it more difficult to maintain a regular exercise schedule.

Appetite control: Thirst is often confused for hunger, which may result in irrational snacking or overeating. Staying hydrated and lowering your chance of mistaking hunger with thirst might help you better control your appetite and consume fewer calories unnecessarily throughout the day.

Supports Digestion: Maintaining regular bowel motions and promoting digestive health both depend on proper water. Water helps facilitate digestion and soften stools, preventing constipation and other discomforts that may result from dehydration. A healthy digestive system is essential for general wellbeing and may aid in your attempts to lose weight.

Recovery and Muscle growth: Staying hydrated is essential for post-workout recovery and muscle growth if you regularly exercise as part of your weight reduction strategy. Water contributes in muscle development and repair by flushing away waste materials and assisting in the delivery of nutrients to your cells. Drinking enough water may boost your workout regimen and encourage the growth of strong muscles.

Remaining Hydrated Advice:

regularly Drink Water Throughout the Day: Make it a point to regularly drink water throughout the day. Keep a water bottle nearby and drink from it often to keep hydrated. Aim for at least 8 to 10 glasses of water each day, or more if the weather is hot or you are physically active.

Hydrate Before and After Exercise: To replace fluids lost via perspiration and promote recuperation, drink water before and after your exercises. Consider consuming sports drinks with electrolytes if you're exercising vigorously or for an extended period of time to help replenish lost minerals like salt, potassium, and magnesium.

Monitor Urine Colour: Your urine's colour might serve as a sign of your level of hydration. While dark yellow or amber-colored urine may suggest dehydration, pale yellow or clear urine often shows appropriate hydration.

Consume hydrating foods: Fruits and vegetables, which have a high water content, may help you stay hydrated all day long. To keep hydrated, include vegetables like cucumbers, melons, oranges, berries, lettuce, and celery in your diet.

Limit your consumption of alcohol and coffee since both substances may dehydrate you. To avoid too diuretic effects, limit your alcohol intake, balance it with water, and decrease your caffeine intake.

Listen to Your Body: When you experience thirst, pay heed to your body's cues and take a sip of water. Don't put off drinking water until you are really thirsty since this might mean that you are already dehydrated.

Always remember to stay hydrated throughout the day, particularly before and after physical activity. Consider include hydrating items in your diet and keeping an eye on the colour of your urine as a sign of your level of hydration. Reduce your consumption of alcohol and caffeine, and pay attention to your body's thirst cues.

You can optimise your body's processes, support your general health, and improve your chances of losing weight by making hydration a priority in your weight reduction strategy. Keep in mind that healthy weight reduction is a slow process, and one of the little but effective lifestyle adjustments you can make to help you along the way is to drink enough of water. So, on your journey to a better, happier self, don't hold back and remain hydrated!

CHAPTER THREE

Building Strong Foundations: Beginner Wall Pilates Exercises

Wall Roll Down for Spinal Mobility and Core Activation

Wall Roll Down is a flexible exercise that combines spinal mobility and core activation. It is simple to add into your exercise regimen and can be modified to accommodate varying degrees of flexibility and fitness. Using the wall as a supporting guide, you may concentrate on maintaining appropriate alignment and form while working on a selected set of muscles.

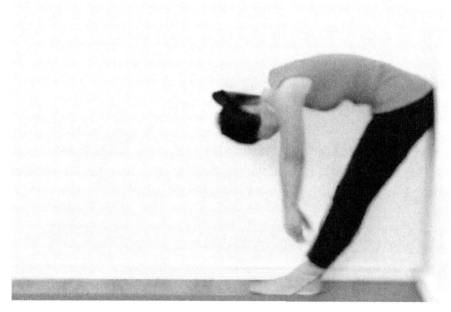

Here is how to go about it:

Step 1: Prepare Your Area

You will need a clean wall area with enough room to stand comfortably with your arms up high before beginning the Wall Roll Down exercise. Make sure the wall is unobstructed and clean. With your feet hip-width apart and your arms straight over your head, take a stance facing the wall. The distance between your heels and the wall should be between 6 and 8 inches, and you should have a neutral spine with your shoulders down.

Step 2: Contract Your Abdomen

It's crucial to contract your core muscles before starting the wall roll down. Start by stimulating your deep abdominal muscles by bringing your navel towards your spine. Try to imagine pulling your belly button inside so that it feels like a corset around your waist. Throughout the workout, this core activation will aid to protect your lower back and stabilise your spine.

Step 3: Start the Movement

Roll down towards the wall while keeping your core engaged and starting to progressively articulate your spine. As you lower your head, neck, upper back, middle back, and lower back towards the wall, start by tucking your chin towards your chest. As you move, keep your shoulders loose and your arms up above. Maintain control and awareness of your body at all times while shifting one vertebra at a time.

Step 4: Feel the stretch

Your spine and the backs of your legs will gradually lengthen as you continue to roll downward. Reach your hands towards the wall and let your body expand and stretch. To preserve your lower back, refrain from any abrupt movements or bouncing and keep your core engaged.

Step 5: Make Wall Contact

Take a moment to catch your breath after your fingers have reached the wall. As you keep your fingers in contact with the wall, notice how your spine is being gently pulled. Your head, shoulders, and hips should all be contacting the wall, and your arms should still be stretched above. Your body should be in a little diagonal posture.

6th step: Roll up

Roll back up to the starting position from the wall contact position. Start the exercise by stomping your feet into the ground, then engage your core and stack your vertebrae back up to a standing posture one at a time. As you roll up, keep your shoulders loose and your arms up above. Maintain control of your body and awareness of each vertebra as you move them.

Step 7: Iterate and Adjust

The Wall Roll Down exercise may be repeated several times once you have finished one session. Attempt 8–10 repetitions, or whichever many you find comfortable. Keep good form, use your core, and move slowly and deliberately during the whole workout. If the exercise is too difficult for you, you may adapt it by bending your knees just a little or by doing it with your back against a wall for more support.

The advantages of wall rolling exercises

The Wall Roll Down exercise has various advantages for improving core strength and spinal mobility. The following are a few of the main advantages of include Wall Roll Down in your Pilates routine:

Spinal Mobility: By articulating the spine's vertebrae one at a time, the Wall Roll Down exercise helps to increase spinal mobility. The whole spine, from the neck to the lower back, is encouraged to be flexible and mobile as a result. Additionally, it aids in easing muscular stiffness and tension in the back, improving posture and lowering the likelihood of back discomfort.

Core Activation: The Wall Roll Down exercise is a fantastic way to engage the deep abdominal muscles, which are essential for stability and strength in Pilates. You may tone your core muscles, including the transverse abdominis, obliques, and pelvic floor muscles, by keeping your core engaged throughout the workout. Enhancing core stability is beneficial for supporting the spine and keeping it in the right position.

Stretching: As you extend your fingers towards the wall during the Wall Roll Down exercise, your spine and the backs of your legs will be stretched. This easy stretch improves flexibility and lessens muscular imbalances by lengthening tight muscles including the hamstrings, calves, and back muscles.

Improved Posture: Sedentary lifestyles and extended sitting contribute to poor posture, which is a widespread problem. The Wall Roll Down exercise encourages optimal alignment of the spine and shoulders, which may aid with posture. Learning to maintain a neutral spine position when you articulate your spine and engage your core will help you maintain improved posture throughout the day and can be applied to daily tasks.

The Pilates method is well renowned for emphasising the link between the mind and body, and the Wall Roll Down exercise is no exception. As you do the exercise, it calls for focus, control, and body awareness. Proprioception, bodily awareness, and mindfulness are all improved as a result, which may promote general wellbeing and mindfulness in other aspects of life.

Exercise with minimal Impact: The Wall Roll Down exercise has a minimal impact and is easy on the joints, making it suited for individuals of all ages and fitness levels. It is the best exercise for those who are recuperating from injuries or have restrictions since it offers a secure and efficient technique to focus on spine mobility and core activation without placing an undue amount of stress on the joints.

Making Wall Roll Downs a Part of Your Pilates Exercises

You may use these instructions to include the Wall Roll Down exercise in your Pilates routine:

Warm-up: It's important to warm up your body before beginning any activity to get it ready for the action. To mobilise the joints and improve blood flow to the muscles, you may execute a warm-up routine that involves moderate motions like neck circles, shoulder rolls, and hip circles.

Set up your area: Locate a spot against a clean wall where you can stand comfortably with your arms up. Make sure the wall is unobstructed and clean.

Activate your deep abdominal muscles and move your navel towards your spine to activate your core before beginning the Wall Roll Down. This aids with spinal stabilisation and lower back protection as you workout.

Observe the detailed directions: The commencement of movement, feeling the stretch, reaching the wall, and rolling back up to the starting position are the first steps in the detailed directions described previously. Focus on articulating your spine one vertebra at a time while moving slowly and deliberately, keeping your core engaged the whole time.

Adjust as necessary: If you find the exercise difficult, you may adjust it by gently bending your knees or by doing it with your back against a wall for more support. Work within your comfort zone while paying attention to your body, gradually increasing the challenge as you advance.

Cool down: To encourage relaxation and recuperation after the Wall Roll Down exercise, you must allow your body to come to room temperature. To alleviate any tension in the muscles and spine, try easy stretches like cat-cow or child's pose.

Regular practise is essential if you want to get the most out of Wall Roll Down as part of your Pilates regimen. For optimum results, add it into your regimen at least twice or three times a week along with other Pilates exercises.

Advice for Practising Wall Roll Downs Effectively

To achieve a good Wall Roll Down exercise, consider the following extra advice:

Remember to breathe: As you reach for the wall and as you roll back up, be mindful of your breath throughout the whole exercise. This supports appropriate mobility, encourages relaxation, and engages the core.

The Wall Roll Down workout requires you to activate your core. Draw your navel towards your spine and maintain a firm core by keeping your deep abdominal muscles engaged throughout the workout.

Move carefully: Instead of speeding through the exercise, concentrate on moving with control and accuracy. Articulate the spine's vertebrae one at a time, staying in control and stable throughout the motion.

Observe your body: During the workout, pay attention to how your body feels and make any necessary adjustments. Stop immediately and change your posture or range of motion if you experience any pain or discomfort. Working inside your comfort zone is crucial in order to prevent pushing yourself above your limits.

Keep your alignment correct: Avoid excessive back rounding or arching during the workout by maintaining your spine in neutral position. Keep your neck in a neutral posture, your shoulders relaxed and away from your ears.

Be patient with yourself. Wall Roll Down may need some practise to perfect. Give yourself time to develop and advance since it's a challenging activity that calls for body awareness, coordination, and control.

Wall Squats

The lower body muscles, such as your quadriceps, hamstrings, glutes, and calves, are the focus of wall squats, often referred to as wall sits. The reason they are known as "Wall Squats" is because they entail maintaining a squatting posture while utilising your body weight as resistance against a wall. This workout is distinctive because it tests your muscles' ability to perform isometrically, or contract and retain a position without moving.

You'll need a strong wall with enough room to lean on it and some open space on the floor in order to execute Wall Squats. Here is a detailed instruction on how to do wall squats:

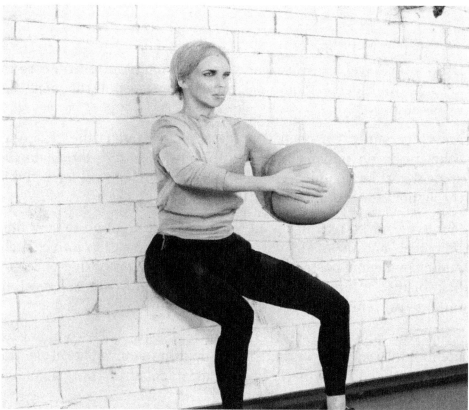

Step 1: Locate a wall and take a stance

Starting position: Stand with your back to a wall, feet hip-width apart, and arms at your sides.

Ensure that your feet are sufficiently far from the wall so that your knees will be squarely over your ankles when you squat.

Step 2: Squat down to the floor.

As you squat down, maintaining your back against the wall, bend your knees and lower your body. Your thighs should be parallel to the floor and your knees should form a 90-degree angle. Keep your feet level on the ground and distribute your weight equally between your heels and your foot's balls.

Step 3: Maintain Your Position

Depending on your degree of comfort and fitness, maintain the squatting posture for a certain period of time. Beginners may begin with 30 seconds and progressively extend it as they gain strength. Maintain good posture by pressing your back into the wall, keeping your abs tight, and keeping your knees in line with your ankles.

Step 4: Stand up again

To stand back up, drive through your heels and contract your glutes and quads. After a brief break, repeat as many times or for as long as desired.

Now that you are familiar with the Wall Squat exercise, let's examine the various advantages of include it in your Pilates routine:

Lower Body Strength: Wall squats are a great workout for developing lower body strength. They concentrate on your calf, glutes, hamstrings, and quadriceps, helping to tone and shape these muscles. Your muscles are functioning isometrically while you maintain the squatting posture against the wall, which may enhance muscular stability and endurance.

Wall squats focus your lower body in particular, but they also work your core muscles. You must use your deep abdominal muscles, particularly your transverse abdominis and obliques, to keep your posture and stability correct. Your overall balance and stability may be improved as a result of strengthening your core.

Wall squats may also aid with joint stability, especially in the hips and knees. You are working the muscles surrounding these joints as you drop into the squatting posture and maintain it against the wall, which improves the stability and support of the joints.

Posture Improvement: Wall squats require that you keep a straight back against the wall, thus good technique is essential. By promoting optimal spinal and pelvic alignment, this may aid in posture improvement. You may experience better posture throughout the day as a result of doing Wall Squats to strengthen your lower body and core muscles.

Flexibility: Wall squats are another exercise that may help you become more flexible, especially in the hips, knees, and ankles. Your muscles and joints are stretched as you drop into the squatting posture, which might eventually result in more flexibility. Your mobility in general and your ability to move freely throughout your day may benefit from this.

Time-efficient: Wall squats are a quick workout that you may do as a stand-alone exercise or as part of your Pilates programme. They may be done anywhere, including at home, the gym, or even the workplace during a fast break since they take up little room and equipment. Wall squats are a practical choice for a busy lifestyle since you can modify their time and intensity to match your level of fitness and schedule.

Progression and variety: Wall squats provide a wide range of progression and variety. Once you've mastered the fundamental Wall Squat, you may add variants to push yourself more and work other muscle groups, such as single-leg Wall Squats, side-to-side Wall Squats, or Wall Squats with a stability ball between your knees. This enables you to advance in your fitness journey by setting new challenges for yourself.

All Fitness Levels may Use Wall Squats: Wall squats may be adjusted to accommodate all fitness levels, making them suitable for both novice and expert exercisers. You may begin with shallower squats if you're new to training or have any physical restrictions, and you can progressively raise the depth as you build strength and confidence. Always pay attention to your body, and if you have any worries or inquiries, speak with a certified fitness expert.

Adding Wall Squats to Your Pilates Exercises

You may be wondering how to include wall squats into your Pilates exercise now that you are aware of their advantages. Here are some pointers to get you going:

right form: Keep your form correct throughout the whole workout. Maintain a tight core, your knees in line with your ankles, and a back against the wall. Keep your back straight and your knees from bending inward. To maintain appropriate technique while doing Wall Squats, you may wish to practise in front of a mirror or with a certified fitness expert.

Gradual development As you grow stronger, progressively extend the time for your Wall Squats from a comfortable starting point, like 30 seconds. To make your squat more difficult over time, you may also add variants or deepen it. Always pay attention to your body's cues and go at your own speed.

As part of a comprehensive Pilates regimen, incorporate: Wall squats are a terrific way to supplement other Pilates exercises that concentrate on core strength, flexibility, and stability in your Pilates regimen. Wall Squats are a great exercise to add to your Pilates regimen along with other moves to target various muscle groups and improve overall fitness.

Rest and recovery: Just as with any activity, it's crucial to allow your muscles some downtime. Avoid doing Wall Squats every day, and give yourself enough time to recover between sets. Pay attention to your body and modify the quantity and force of your Wall Squats as necessary.

Wall Leg Press for Glute Activation and Leg Toning

A flexible and dynamic exercise, the wall leg press works your glutes, hamstrings, quadriceps, and calves while also taxing your stability and core. Maintaining perfect form and control while lifting your legs up against a wall helps to tone your legs and engage your glutes.

The ability of the Wall Leg Press to engage and build your glute muscles is one of its key advantages. The three muscles that make up your glutes—the gluteus maximus, gluteus medius, and gluteus minimus—are the biggest and strongest in your body. They are essential for numerous functional motions, like squatting, jogging, and walking. They also give your buttocks a hard, toned look.

Wall Leg Press stimulates your hamstrings, which are the muscles at the back of your thighs, in addition to activating your glutes. Hamstrings that are toned and strong not only give your legs a balanced, sculpted look, but they also increase the stability and strength of the whole lower body.

The quadriceps, which are the muscles at the front of your thighs and are in charge of knee extension and leg strength, are also activated by the Wall Leg Press. Quadriceps that are well-toned not only make your legs seem better, but they help support your knees and make your motions more functional.

The muscles on the rear of your lower legs known as the calves are also worked out with the Wall Leg Press. with addition to helping to balance the look of the legs, calves that are strong and toned also aid with ankle stability and general lower body strength.

How to Do a Wall Leg Press Properly

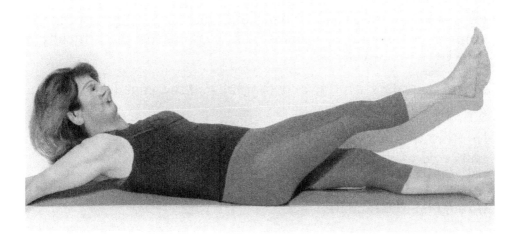

It's essential to carry out the Wall Leg Press exercise with appropriate form in order to get the most out of it and prevent injuries. Here is a step-by-step explanation on how to do the Wall Leg Press properly:

Locate a wall with no obstructions: Decide on a wall where you have room to comfortably stretch your legs. Make sure the wall is unobstructed and clean.

With your feet hip-width apart and your toes pointed forward, take a stance facing the wall. For support, place your hands at shoulder height on the wall.

Draw your belly button towards your spine and tighten the muscles in your core to keep yourself stable while you do the exercise.

Lean back and push your legs up against the wall: Press your legs up against the wall while slowly leaning back and maintaining your feet on the ground. Your heels should be firmly planted on the wall, and your knees should be slightly bent.

Legs extended: Slowly straighten your legs and firmly place them against the wall. Throughout the exercise, maintain a neutral spine and a tight core.

Hold for a few seconds, then gradually release the posture by bending your knees and bringing your feet back to the beginning position.

Repeat as many times as needed: Exercise for the appropriate number of repetitions, progressively stepping up the difficulty as your strength improves.

Keep your spine neutral and prevent curving your lower back as part of proper form.

In order to prevent hyperextension, keep your knees slightly bent and avoid pressing too firmly against the wall.

To maximise glute activation, hold your heels firmly on the wall throughout the exercise.

As you lean your legs up against the wall, concentrate on your breathing by taking a deep breath in and an exhale as you let go.

Start with a modest degree of difficulty and progressively up the ante by extending the time of the hold or straightening your legs more as you gain strength.

Including Wall Leg Presses in Your Pilates Exercise Programme

In order to focus your glutes and tone your legs, adding the Wall Leg Press to your Pilates programme might be beneficial. The following advice will help you include the wall leg press in your Pilates routine:

Warm-up: To get your muscles and joints ready for the workout, warm-up before any activity. An easy aerobic workout for a few minutes, such brisk walking or cycling, may be followed by some dynamic stretches for your hips, legs, and core.

Leg Press on a Wall: Apply the Wall Leg Press as previously taught, paying close attention to form and control. As you gain stronger, progressively up the challenge level from moderate to intense.

variants: You may attempt many Wall Leg Press variants to spice up and challenge your practise. For increased resistance, you might add ankle weights or execute the exercise with one leg at a time while maintaining the other leg in a tabletop position.

Exercises that go along with the Wall Leg Press include Pilates moves that work your glutes, legs, and core. For a whole lower body workout, the Wall Leg Press may be combined with exercises like Pilates bridges, leg circles, and clams.

Cool-down: After your Pilates exercise, stretch and relax your muscles with a cool-down. For your glutes, hamstrings, quadriceps, and calves, you may do static stretches and hold each one for 15 to 30 seconds.

The Advantages of Wall Leg Press for Leg Toning and Glute Activation

Your fitness journey may benefit greatly from adding Wall Leg Press to your Pilates programme. The following are some of the main advantages of Wall Leg Press:

Wall Leg Press is a very powerful workout for engaging and enlarging your glutes. Your glute muscles are worked by pushing up against the wall, which helps lift and tone your buttocks and give them a hard, sculpted look.

Strengthening and toning your legs: The Wall Leg Press works your hamstrings, quadriceps, and calves. Your lower body will look better if your legs are toned, and they will also improve your functional motions and general lower body strength.

Engaging your core muscles is necessary for the Wall Leg Press in order to maintain stability and control. This aids in strengthening your core, which is necessary for general stability, posture, and practical everyday movement.

Convenience: Because Wall Leg Press can be done anyplace there is a clean wall area, it is a handy exercise that can be quickly included into your Pilates programme or performed on its own when you don't have access to gym equipment or have limited time.

Versatility: Wall Leg Press is versatile in terms of variants and degrees of difficulty. You may adapt the workout to your fitness level and objectives by starting with a moderate degree of difficulty and progressively moving to more challenging variants as you gain stronger.

Wall Bridge for Core Stability and Glute Strengthening

Let's first examine the benefits of core stability and glute strengthening for general health and fitness before delving into the specifics of the Wall Bridge exercise.

The capacity to keep your spine and pelvis in a solid and balanced posture while moving is referred to as core stability. An efficient core supports good posture, lowers injury risk, and supports effective movement in sports and daily activities. Your spine is stabilised and supported by the core muscles, which include the deep abdominal muscles, back muscles, and pelvic floor muscles.

Your glutes, on the other hand, the muscles in your buttocks, are very important for hip extension, rotation, and stabilisation. For functional motions like walking, jogging, and lifting, strong glutes are necessary. They may also aid with posture and lower back pain relief.

Let's now examine how the Wall Bridge exercise might aid in strengthening your core and glutes.

A wall provides additional support for the Wall Bridge exercise, which is a modification of the traditional Pilates bridge exercise. Beginners and those with restricted mobility may execute the workout on it since it offers a sturdy platform. The following are a few advantages of the Wall Bridge exercise:

Improve core stability by using your deep abdominal muscles, back muscles, and pelvic floor muscles with the Wall Bridge exercise. Additionally, it encourages optimal spinal alignment, which is necessary for a healthy back and excellent posture.

The Wall Bridge exercise works your glutes especially, helping to tone and develop these muscles. It engages the gluteus medius, a smaller muscle on the outside of your buttocks, as well as the gluteus maximus, the biggest muscle in your buttocks. Your balance, lower body strength, and hip stability may all be enhanced by having strong glutes.

Muscles at the back of your thighs known as the hamstrings are also activated during the Wall Bridge exercise. You may enhance your knee stability and avoid hamstring problems by strengthening your hamstrings.

Let's now review the appropriate form for doing the Wall Bridge exercise:

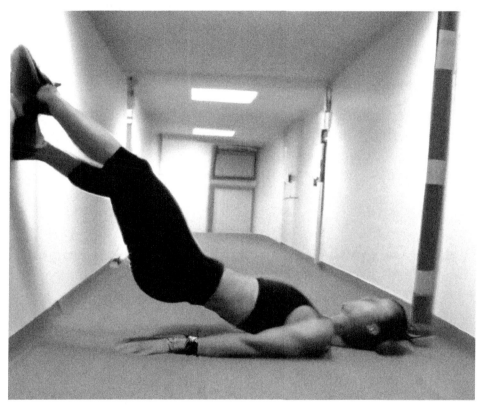

Lay on your back with your feet hip-width apart and your knees bent at a 90-degree angle against a clean wall. By your sides, your arms should be at ease.

Your core should be engaged by bringing your navel towards your spine while you firmly plant your feet on the wall.

Keeping your feet firmly planted on the wall, slowly raise your hips off the mat and towards the ceiling. Your hips, shoulders, and knees need to be in a straight line.

After a brief period of holding the bridge posture, carefully bring your hips back to the mat.

Repeat for 10 to 15 times, paying close attention to your form and control at all times.

Tips for Proper Form: To maximise glute and hamstring activation, keep your feet firmly planted on the wall throughout the exercise.

To avoid straining your lower back, try not to lift your hips too high. From your knees to your shoulders, try to form a straight line.

To maintain stability and safeguard your lower back during the workout, engage your core by pulling your navel towards your spine.

Throughout the exercise, breathe normally, taking in air as you drop your hips and exhaling as you elevate them.

Including the Wall Bridge in Your Pilates Exercises

Let's look at how to include the Wall Bridge exercise in your Pilates programme so you can benefit from it now that you know how to do it correctly.

Warm-up: Warm-up your body before beginning any activity to improve blood flow, loosen up your muscles, and get ready for the workout. After doing some mild aerobic workouts like brisk walking or cycling, you may stretch your hips, hamstrings, and lower back dynamically.

As a stand-alone exercise, Wall Bridge: The Wall Bridge exercise may be done independently as part of your Pilates regimen. Focus on good technique and control as you begin with 1-2 sets of 10-15 repetitions. You may progressively boost the number of sets or repetitions as you gain stronger and more at ease.

Including additional exercises: For a more difficult and dynamic workout, the Wall Bridge exercise may be combined with other

Pilates moves. To effectively target your core, glutes, and thighs, you may pair it with exercises like the single-leg bridge, scissor, or Pilates toe taps. To prevent overexertion or strain, constantly remember to maintain appropriate form and control and pay attention to your body.

Progression and modification options: There are a number of ways you may advance or alter the Wall Bridge exercise. To enhance the difficulty and further work your glutes and core, consider raising one leg off the wall while executing the exercise. To increase the difficulty and intensity of the workout, you may also place an exercise ball or a Pilates ring in between your thighs. Before advancing or changing the workout, ensure sure you're comfortable and able to maintain appropriate form.

Wall Abdominal Curls for Core Activation and Abdominal Toning

The rectus abdominis, or "six-pack" muscles, are the focus of the Pilates exercise known as wall abdominal curls, often referred to as wall curls or wall roll-ups. The goal of this exercise is to curl your upper body towards your knees while keeping your feet firmly planted on the wall. To do it, lie on your back with your feet up against a wall. Though it may seem straightforward at first, this workout is quite intense and highly effective.

The ability to engage the deep core muscles, such as the transverse abdominis and the pelvic floor muscles, is one of the main advantages of wall abdominal curls. These muscles are essential for supporting and stabilising the spine, enhancing posture, and avoiding lower back discomfort. You may build a strong and stable core by working these muscles using wall abdominal curls, which acts as a firm base for subsequent workouts and motions.

The ability of wall abdominal curls to tone the abdominal muscles is another benefit. This workout targets the rectus abdominis, the superficial muscle that gives the illusion of a "six-pack". Wall Abdominal Curls will assist you in gaining a distinct stomach and a toned body by using controlled and exact motions, which will improve your entire physique and appearance.

Let's now examine the Wall Abdominal Curl method in more detail. To successfully complete this exercise, adhere to the following step-by-step directions:

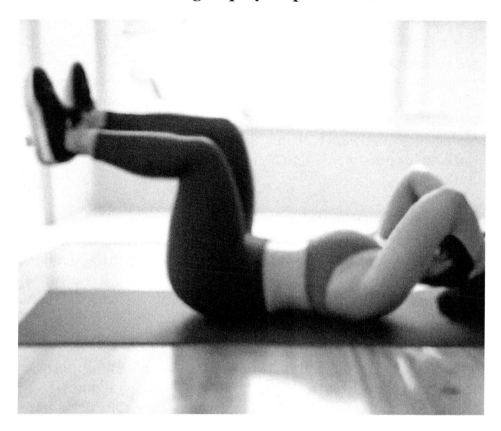

Locate a spot away from a wall, then lay on your back with your arms at your sides. Place your feet on the wall with your knees bent and your feet hip-width apart with your toes pointed upward.

Inhale deeply, then get ready to tighten your core. Start peeling one vertebra at a time as you start to curl your upper body off the mat as you exhale. To prevent straining your neck, picture extending your chest towards your knees while keeping your chin tucked in close to your chest.

Maintaining a C-curve with your spine, curl up farther until you are at a comfortable height. Hold this posture for a short period of time while feeling your abdominal muscles tense.

Take a deep breath in and controllably drop your upper body back down, articulating your spine one vertebra at a time. After the required amount of repetitions, go back to where you were before and repeat.

To guarantee the exercise's greatest efficiency and avoid injuries, it's crucial to keep your form and alignment correct the whole time. Focus on utilising your core muscles to begin and control the action rather than swinging your body or using momentum. Before starting any new fitness programme, it is always advisable to speak with a certified Pilates teacher or healthcare provider, especially if you are new to the discipline or have any pre-existing health issues.

Let's now examine several Wall Abdominal Curl variants you may use to spice up and challenge your routine:

Abdominal wall curls with one leg only: With one leg stretched towards the sky and the other foot firmly planted on the wall, do the Wall Abdominal Curls. This version ups the difficulty and calls for greater control and stability from your core muscles.

Curls of the oblique abdominal wall: Reach your opposing shoulder towards your opposite knee as you bend your knees and shift your torso to one side. To work the oblique muscles, which are in charge of side waist definition, alternate sides throughout each exercise.

Beginning with both legs extended towards the sky, do scissor wall abdominal curls by lowering one leg to the floor and curling your upper body towards the knee of the other leg. For a hard exercise, alternate sides throughout each repeat to engage both your upper and lower abs.

Knee Tucks: If you want, you may maintain your feet firmly planted on the wall and pull your knees to your chest instead of curling your upper body towards your knees. This version increases the difficulty of your core exercise by focusing on the hip flexors in addition to the rectus abdominis.

By using these variations in your routine, you can give your Wall Abdominal Curls more variety and difficulty, which will help you advance and keep building core strength and abdominal tone.

Here are some helpful pointers to keep in mind while doing Wall Abdominal Curls to maximise its effectiveness and guarantee the best results:

Focus on Quality Over Quantity: Performing Wall Abdominal Curls with good form and control is preferable than speeding through the exercise with subpar technique, even if you can only complete a few repetitions. In order to activate the proper muscles and avoid injuries, movement quality is essential.

Activate Your Core Focus on using your deep core muscles, such as the transverse abdominis and the pelvic floor muscles, during the whole exercise. Instead of grabbing your hip flexors, shoulders, or neck, utilise your core to start and control the action.

Breathe Efficiently: In all Pilates exercises, including Wall Abdominal Curls, proper breathing is essential. Exhale as you curl up and pull your navel towards your spine after taking a deep breath to become ready. To come back down safely, inhale. You may strengthen your connection to your core and increase the efficacy of the workout by taking slow, deep breaths.

Gradually proceed to more difficult varieties as you build strength and control. If you are new to Pilates or Wall Abdominal Curls in general, start with the simpler variety. It's important to advance safely and steadily, so pay attention to your body and don't push yourself above your limitations.

CHAPTER FOUR

Taking It to the Next Level: Intermediate Wall Pilates Exercises

Wall Scissor for Leg Toning and Abdominal Activation

The standard Pilates Scissor exercise, which is often done on a mat, is modified by the Wall Scissor exercise. The wall offers additional stability and support, enabling you to concentrate on successfully using certain muscle groups. The quadriceps, hamstrings, and inner thighs are the main muscles that this exercise targets in your legs. It also activates your core by working your deep abdominal muscles. It is a fantastic workout for increasing body awareness, flexibility, and strength.

To perform the Wall Scissor exercise, follow these steps:

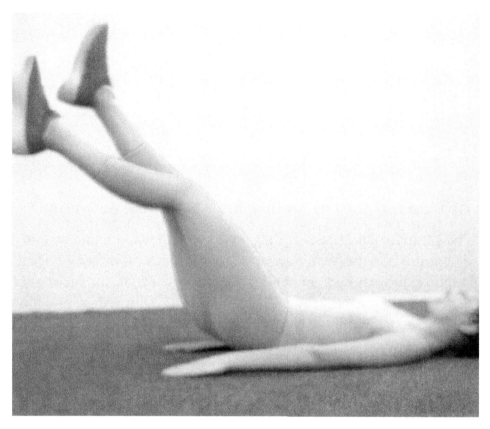

Step 1: Preparation

Lay down against a wall that is free of obstructions, with your arms at your sides and your legs stretched upward.

With your toes pointed upward, lean your heels up against the wall. Your legs have to be parallel to the floor and straight, making a 90-degree angle with the wall.

Draw your navel towards your spine to activate your core, and tuck your lower back into the mat.

Step 2: Movement

Prepare by taking a deep breath in, then gently drop one leg towards the floor while maintaining its straightness and keeping it a few inches above the ground. Lift the opposite leg at the same time, maintaining it parallel to the floor and firmly pushing it against the wall.

Taking a breath in, carefully drop the lifted leg towards the floor while raising the other leg towards the ceiling to change legs. Throughout the workout, keep your movements controlled and precise while keeping your legs straight and using your core.

For 8 to 10 repetitions on each leg, or as many as you can manage while maintaining perfect form and control, repeat the scissor-like motions.

Safety Advice

To maximise the benefits and reduce the danger of injury, it's critical to pay close attention to your form and technique when you execute the Wall Scissor exercise. Observe the following advice:

Maintain focus at your centre: Focus on bringing your navel towards your spine and keeping your pelvis neutral and steady throughout the exercise. Your lower back and deep abdominal muscles will also benefit from this.

Keep your alignment: Legs should be pressed firmly against the wall while remaining straight and parallel to the floor. Keep your motions regulated and precise, and try not to bend or twist your legs.

Manage your breathing: Exhale as you drop your leg towards the floor after taking a deep breath to prepare. Taking a second breath, swap legs. To improve your control and stability, sync your breath with your motions.

Observe your body: If you experience any pain or tension in your neck, hips, or lower back, adapt the exercise or, if necessary, stop. To avoid injuries, it's critical to respect your body's limitations and operate within your comfort zone.

Variations and modifications

After learning the proper technique for the Wall Scissor exercise, let's look at several adjustments and variants to make it more difficult or appropriate for people of different fitness levels.

Resistance band and wall scissors: You may add another level of difficulty to the workout by wrapping a resistance band around your feet and securing it to the wall behind you. With the addition of resistance from the resistance band, the leg motions become more difficult and involve more muscles in your legs and core. As you become stronger and more used to the workout, gradually increase the resistance by starting with a lighter resistance band.

Wall Scissor with Leg Circles: Adding leg circles to the Wall Scissor exercise is another variant. While maintaining the other leg pressed up against the wall, drop one leg to the floor and begin circling it. Halfway through the repetitions, switch the circles' directions. This version puts more strain on your hip flexors and outer thighs while posing an additional test to your core stability.

Wall Scissor with Extended Arms: While completing the Wall Scissor exercise, you may extend your arms upward to further activate your upper body. In this variant, you must maintain your upper body stability while moving your legs, which adds a level of coordination and balance. Additionally, it strengthens your upper back, arms, and shoulders while testing your shoulder stability.

Wall Scissor with Bent Knee: You may adjust this exercise by bending your knees just a little bit if you find the straight-leg posture too difficult or unpleasant. With this adjustment, you can pay attention to activating your core and keeping your alignment correct without putting too much pressure on your lower back. You may progressively straighten your legs to increase the difficulty as you become more comfortable.

The advantages of wall scissors

Numerous advantages of the Wall Scissor workout include leg toning and abdominal activation. The following are some major benefits of include this exercise in your Pilates routine:

Leg toning: The Wall Scissor exercise works the quadriceps, hamstrings, and inner thighs of your legs. These muscles are sculpted and toned by the regulated and exact actions, resulting in slimmer and stronger legs.

Core Activation: To maintain stability and control during the Wall Scissor exercise, you must contract your deep abdominal muscles. Your transverse abdominis, rectus abdominis, and obliques are all strengthened as a result, which improves core stability and posture.

Increased Flexibility: As you lower and elevate your legs during the Wall Scissor exercise, your hamstrings and hip flexors are stretched and lengthened. This exercise may help you become more flexible in these regions over time, giving you more range of motion in your hips and legs.

Body Awareness: The Wall Scissor exercise improves body awareness by requiring you to pay attention to your alignment, breath, and body posture. This increased awareness may be applied to other everyday tasks, encouraging improved posture, efficient movement, and injury avoidance.

Challenge and Variation: You may adjust the Wall Scissor workout to meet your fitness level and objectives thanks to its many adjustments and variants. Resistance bands, leg circles, or extended arms may make the exercise more difficult, offering possibilities for advancement and ongoing growth.

Wall Teaser for Core Strengthening and Balance

The Pilates training mainstay known as the Teaser exercise has a new version known as the Wall Teaser. The Wall Teaser, on the other hand, is done with the assistance of a wall, bringing an additional element of stability and control to the exercise.

To perform the Wall Teaser, follow these steps:

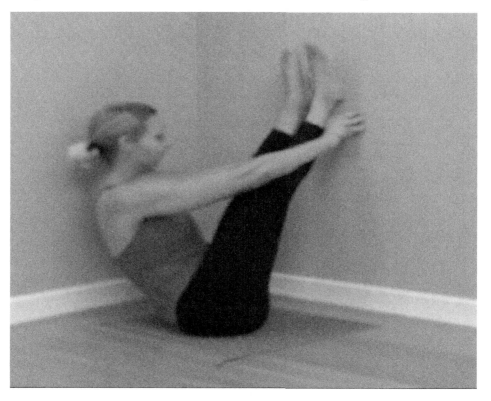

Find a spot against a clean wall, lean against it with your back, and sit with your legs out in front of you. Your arms should be straight out in front of you, parallel to the floor, and your feet should be hip-width apart.

Roll down through your spine gradually, maintaining your back against the wall, until your legs are fully stretched and you are laying on the ground. Your arms should be aloft and resting on the floor while your feet should be pressed on the wall.

Exhale as you pull your spine up off the floor one vertebra at a time, engaging your core as you do so. Continue until you are sitting up in a V shape with your legs still extended and your arms reaching towards your feet.

Exhale after you gently roll back down through your spine, retaining control and keeping your back against the wall, until you are resting on the floor once again. Inhale to hold the posture.

Repeat the exercise as many times as necessary.

Benefits

Now that you know how to do the Wall Teaser, let's examine the advantages it may provide for your balance and core muscles:

Strengthening the core: The Wall Teaser is an effective exercise that focuses on the deep abdominal muscles, obliques, and lower back muscles, all of which are significant parts of the core. The Wall Teaser may assist you in developing a solid and stable core while working these muscles, which will enhance your posture, balance, and overall level of functional fitness.

Balance & Stability: As you roll up into a V shape and hold the posture, the Wall Teaser tests your balance and stability. Your core must be engaged, your stabilising muscles must be engaged, and you must maintain control throughout the exercise. Over time, this may assist in enhancing your stability and balance in both your regular activities and your Pilates practise.

Flexibility and mobility are also necessary for the Wall Teaser since it works your spine, hips, and shoulders. You must slide through these joints with ease and control as you roll up and down. Your flexibility and mobility may be enhanced with regular practise of the Wall Teaser, enabling you to move more effectively throughout your day.

Improved Posture: Good posture is essential for general health and wellness. The Wall Teaser exhorts you to maintain an upright stance with your shoulders relaxed and your spine stretched. You may improve your everyday posture by repeating good posture habits while exercising, which will help you stand taller and move with better alignment.

Like other Pilates exercises, the Wall Teaser emphasises the mind-body link and calls for your full attention to your posture, breath, and movement patterns. Better body awareness, mindfulness, and focus may result from doing this, and they can spread to other aspects of your life as well.

Wall Teaser Integration into Your Pilates Practise

Here are some pointers to keep in mind if you want to include the Wall Teaser into your Pilates routine:

Start with adjustments: It's crucial to start with modifications if you're new to the Wall Teaser or if you have any physical restrictions. You may support yourself by bending your knees or placing a small towel or yoga block under your head. You may progressively advance to the exercise's full expression as your strength and control increase.

Focus on alignment: With the Wall Teaser, alignment is essential to ensuring that you're working the proper muscles and getting the most out of the exercise. To maintain a steady and controlled stance, keep your back pushed up against the wall the whole time. Avoid hunching your shoulders or arching your spine.

Be aware of your breathing while you complete the Wall Teaser. Exhale as you roll up and down after inhaling to become ready. To support the motion and contract your deep abdominal muscles, breathe. Refrain from holding your breath or taking short breaths.

Be persistent and patient: The Wall Teaser may be difficult, and it could take some time to develop the strength and control enough to execute it without effort. To observe improvement, practise often and with patience towards oneself. Always pay attention to your body's signals and go at your own speed.

Add variety: After you've mastered the fundamental Wall Teaser, you can mix up your practise by looking at several tweaks and variants. Try side-lying Wall Teasers, where you execute the exercise while laying on your side, or single-leg Wall Teasers, where you elevate one leg off the ground. These changes may make your practise more interesting and engaging while also testing your balance and core further.

Your core strengthening and balance training may gain a dynamic and useful aspect by including the Wall Teaser into your Pilates regimen. The Wall Teaser has several advantages that may improve your overall fitness and wellness since it places a strong emphasis on alignment, stability, and mind-body connection.

Take advantage of a blank wall area, roll over to your mat, and attempt the Wall Teaser. You could experience better posture, balance, and core strength with time and effort, as well as more diversity and difficulty in your Pilates routine. Prepare to use the Wall Teaser to take your Pilates practise to new heights!

Wall Swan for Spinal Mobility and Upper Body Toning

The Pilates exercise known as the Wall Swan encourages spinal mobility and tones the upper body muscles by using a wall as a support. This exercise is a modification of the traditional Swan exercise, which is often done on a mat. All fitness levels, including novices and those with restricted mobility, may do the Wall Swan since it adds more support and stability.

This workout engages the core muscles and encourages appropriate spinal alignment while also focusing on the upper back, shoulders, and arm muscles. It is a flexible exercise that can be tailored to meet specific requirements and objectives, making it an important component of any Pilates regimen.

Benefits of the Wall Swan

The Wall Swan has a lot of health and fitness-related advantages. The following are some major benefits of include this exercise in your Pilates routine:

A healthier and more functioning spine may be maintained through improving spinal mobility, which is a goal of The Wall Swan. It improves posture by encouraging flexibility and mobility in the spine as well as stretching and strengthening the muscles of the upper back.

Strengthening and toning of the upper body: The Wall Swan focuses on the muscles in the upper back, shoulders, and arms. This exercise, when performed often, may enhance posture, upper body strength, and muscular tone.

Core Engagement: The Wall Swan works the core muscles, including the deep abdominal muscles and the muscles of the pelvic floor, much as other Pilates exercises do. This aids in strengthening the core, which is necessary for general fitness and practical mobility.

Postural Alignment: Maintaining excellent posture and avoiding postural imbalances need proper spinal alignment. The Wall Swan encourages optimal spinal, shoulder, and pelvic alignment, which will improve your daily posture and alignment awareness.

Pilates is renowned for emphasising the mind-body connection, and the Wall Swan is no different. By requiring attention, focus, and control throughout this exercise, you may improve your body awareness and mindfulness while doing Pilates.

How to Perform the Wall Swan

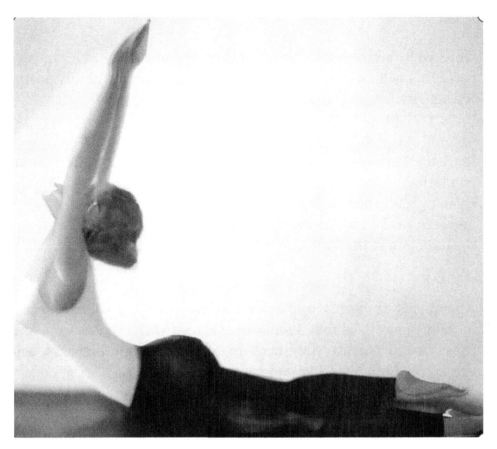

Now that you are aware of the advantages of the Wall Swan exercise, let's examine how to do it correctly. To get started, do these actions:

Set up: Locate a spot against a clean wall where you can lay down comfortably with your arms outstretched. For support, put a small towel folded in half or a pillow under your head. Your toes should be contacting the wall while you are lying on your stomach with your legs straight behind you.

Put your hands shoulder-width apart on the ground with your fingers pointed in the direction of the wall. Your shoulders should be relaxed away from your ears, and your elbows should be slightly bent.

Draw your navel towards your spine to activate the muscles in your core. This will assist you in maintaining control and stability during the activity.

Start the Movement: Take a deep breath to warm up, and then as you exhale, push into your hands and raise your chest off the ground, gently bending your spine. Imagine maintaining your pelvis and legs relaxed while moving your breastbone up and forward in the direction of the wall.

Rhomboids, trapezius, and erector spinae are some of the muscles in your upper back that should be engaged when you elevate your chest. Avoid tensing your neck or squeezing your buttocks, and keep your shoulders loose and away from your ears.

Maintain Control: Hold the raised posture for a few breaths while keeping your upper and lower body stable and in control. Keep your chin parallel to the floor and your forward look.

With a controlled inhalation, drop your chest back to the ground while keeping your spine in the right position. Focus on making controlled and fluid motions as you do the action for the necessary amount of repetitions.

Advice on How to Include the Wall Swan in Your Pilates Routine

Here are some suggestions to keep in mind so that you may get the most out of your Wall Swan exercise:

Start with a Modified Version: You may begin with a modified version of the Wall Swan if you are new to Pilates or have restricted spinal mobility. To lessen the exercise's range of motion and intensity, raise your hands up higher on the wall so they are closer to your shoulders. Work your way down the wall gradually as you become stronger and more flexible.

Remember to use your core muscles throughout the workout by bringing your navel towards your spine. By doing so, you'll be able to keep your balance and control and save your lower back any needless stress.

Focus on Movement Quality: Pay attention to the quality of your movements rather than hurrying through the workout. Consider your alignment and muscle engagement as you move gently and steadily. This will enable you to benefit fully from the workout and lower your risk of suffering an injury.

Breathe Mindfully: Pilates places a strong emphasis on conscious breathing, so be sure to inhale and exhale thoroughly at all times. Keep your body and mind in sync by controlling and initiating your actions with your breath.

Include variants: Once you're familiar with the fundamental Wall Swan exercise, you may experiment with several variants to increase the diversity and complexity of your Pilates routine. To further work your upper body muscles, consider raising one leg off the floor while maintaining the backbend posture or adding brief pulses at the peak of the action

Wall Side Leg Lifts for Hip Strengthening and Toning

The glutes, outer thighs, and hip abductors are the primary muscles of the hips that are used during the difficult exercise known as wall side leg lifts. A wall may be used during this exercise to give stability and aid in maintaining perfect form.

Here's how to perform wall side leg lifts:

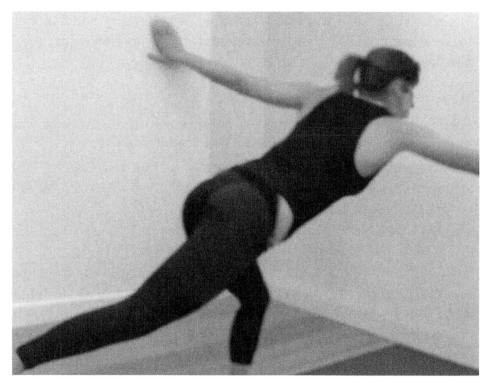

Set up: Place yourself about an arm's length away from a wall with your side towards it. Make sure your feet are hip-width apart and place one hand on the wall for support. Maintain a neutral spine with a little, natural curvature in your lower back while engaging your core.

Lift the Leg: While keeping your body straight and your abs tight, lift one leg, beginning with the heel, towards the direction of the wall. Keep your toes pointed forward and your foot flexed. Do not tilt your pelvis or arch your back.

Control the Movement: Pay attention to regulating the movement as you elevate your leg and keeping it in the right position. Avoid twisting or tilting your hips, and keep them stacked. Avoiding any pain or discomfort, raise your leg to a comfortable height.

Lower Controllably: Carefully lower your leg back down, keeping your hips in their natural position. Refrain from dropping your leg or bending at the hip when standing.

Repetition: Perform the exercise as many times as you'd like, and then switch to the other side.

Benefits of Leg Lifts on the Wall-Side

Leg raises against the wall provide several advantages for hip strengthening and toning. Among the main advantages are:

Strengthened Hips: Wall side leg lifts focus on the hip muscles, especially the glutes, outer thighs, and hip abductors, which helps to strengthen and stabilise the hip joint.

Improved Hip Mobility: By putting the muscles that govern hip abduction, or the movement of the leg away from the midline of the body, to the test, this exercise also helps to enhance hip mobility.

Enhanced Core Engagement: Wall side leg raises, like the majority of Pilates exercises, call for the transverse abdominis and pelvic floor muscles to be properly engaged. This helps to increase core stability and strength.

Better Balance and Stability: Wall side leg lifts may enhance your general balance and proprioception, or your body's knowledge of its location in space, by testing your balance and stability.

Outer thighs and hips may be toned and sculpted with regular practise of wall side leg lifts, which will give your lower body a more defined and toned appearance.

Advice for Correct Form

Here are some suggestions to make sure your wall side leg lifts are safe and efficient and that you are completing them with appropriate form:

Keep Your Body In good Alignment: Throughout the workout, keep your body in good alignment. Do not tilt your pelvis, rotate your hips, or arch your back. Keep your spine neutral and your core active.

Focus on Control: Pay close attention to how the movement is controlled, both going up and going down. Use the muscles in your hip and outer thigh to steadily raise and lower your leg instead of swinging or jerking it.

Keep Your Foot Flexed: Throughout the workout, keep your foot flexed with your toes facing forward. This makes it easier to efficiently contract the hip abductors and outer thigh muscles.

Avoid elevating your leg too high; instead, raise it to a level that is comfortable and pain-free. Avoid elevating your leg too high or pushing it beyond what feels comfortable for your body. Movement quality is more significant than movement volume.

Breathe: Throughout the activity, don't forget to breathe. As you raise your leg, inhale; as you lower it, exhale. Continue to breathe normally and easily.

Use the Wall as Support: The wall is there to provide support, so take use of that fact. Put a gentle hand on the wall to assist you stay stable and in balance, but try not to depend on it too much. The idea is to execute the manoeuvre using your hip muscles.

Increase Difficulty progressively: If you find wall side leg lifts to be too easy, you may progressively toughen them up by adding ankle weights or encircling your ankles with a resistance band. This might increase the difficulty and help to further develop your hip muscles.

Including Wall Side Leg Lifts in Your Pilates Exercise Programme

In particular, if you want to increase hip strength and tone your hips and outer thighs, wall side leg lifts might be a useful addition to your Pilates programme. Following are some pointers for including wall side leg raises in your Pilates routine:

Warm-up: To get your body ready for activity, you should warm up before beginning any workout. Gently moving exercises like pelvic tilts, hip circles, and cat-cow stretches will help you warm up your hips, pelvis, and lower back in a short amount of time.

Start with the Right Alignment: Stand an arm's length away from the wall with your side towards it. Make sure your feet are hip-width apart and place a gentle hand on the wall for support. Keep your spine neutral with a tiny natural curvature in your lower back while engaging your core and relaxing your shoulders.

Start with a Few Repetitions: If you're new to wall side leg lifts, start with a few repetitions on each side. As you become more comfortable with the exercise, you may progressively increase the amount of repetitions. Movement quality is more significant than movement volume.

Focus on Control and Form: Pay attention to regulating the action and maintaining good form while you complete wall side leg raises. Keep your foot flexed with your toes pointed forward and avoid hurrying or jerking your leg. Be mindful of your breathing, core involvement, and alignment.

Gradually increase the difficulty by employing a resistance band around your ankles or adding ankle weights after you are familiar with the basic form of wall side leg lifts. Make sure the resistance you choose will make you work harder without affecting your form.

As with any workout, it's vital to pay attention to your body. If you experience any pain or discomfort, you should adapt your activity or stop altogether. Because every person's body is unique, respect your own limits and go forward at your own speed.

Stretch your hip muscles, outer thighs, and lower back for a few minutes after doing your wall-side leg lifts as a cool-down exercise.

Please keep writing to let out any tension and aid with muscle rehabilitation. Increase flexibility and lessen muscular pain by doing gentle stretches including hip flexor, piriformis, and forward folds.

CHAPTER FIVE

Challenging Your Body: Advanced Wall Pilates Exercises

Wall Pike for Core Strength and Upper Body Toning

The traditional Pike exercise, a mainstay of Pilates and other fitness specialties, has a version called Wall Pike. It incorporates a controlled motion that works the muscles in the upper back, shoulders, and arms. With the feet against the wall when doing the Wall Pike, the exercise is made more difficult and the workout is made harder.

Benefits of Wall Pike

Wall Pike is an excellent addition to any exercise regimen because of its many advantages. Here are a few of the main advantages:

Core Strength: The abdominals, obliques, and lower back are among the core muscles that Wall Pike predominantly targets. The deliberate motion of elevating the hips towards the wall engages the core muscles strongly, promoting core stability and strength.

Wall Pike works the muscles in the upper body, including as the shoulders, arms, and upper back, in addition to the core. A more defined upper body is the consequence of the weight-bearing aspect of the exercise against the wall, which provides resistance and tones and strengthens these muscles.

Better Posture: Maintaining neutral spinal alignment and good posture are essential components of the Wall Pike exercise. By encouraging optimal alignment and strengthening the muscles that maintain healthy posture, this exercise may aid in posture improvement.

Increased Flexibility: In order to do Wall Pike with control, you need to be more flexible in your hamstrings, hips, and lower back. Increased range of motion and more overall flexibility may result from regular Wall Pike practise, which can aid to build flexibility in these regions.

The balance and stability needed to do Wall Pike against a wall tests the muscles in the core and the stabilisers. This may eventually aid in enhancing balance and stability, two things needed for a variety of physical exercises and daily motions.

How to Perform Wall Pike

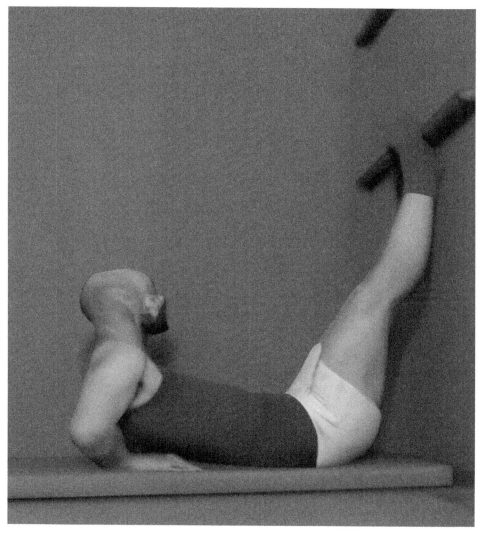

Here is a detailed explanation on how to do Wall Pike:

Locate a free wall space: Look for a wall area that is free of any obstacles and has enough space for you to comfortably do the exercise.

Start in the plank position: Place your feet on the wall and your hands shoulder-width apart on the floor. Your shoulders should be squarely above your wrists, your core should be engaged, and your body should be in a straight line from head to heels.

Slowly raise your hips towards the wall while maintaining your legs straight and your feet pressed up on the structure. Your shoulders should still be over your wrists as your body forms an inverted V.

Maintaining good form and alignment throughout the action, bring your hips back down to the beginning plank posture with control.

Repeat for desired amount of reps, paying close attention to controlled motions and keeping appropriate form.

Advice on How to Perform Wall Pike

Following are some pointers for doing Wall Pike:

Start with adjustments: To make the workout simpler for beginners, start with adjustments. To make the exercise easier, you may, for instance, start with a limited range of motion or place your feet higher up on the wall while doing it.

Keep your attention on form and control: When doing the Wall Pike, proper form and control are crucial. Engage your core, keep your spine neutral, and refrain from overarching or rounding your back. Instead than concentrating on speed or the number of repetitions, move slowly and with control, emphasising the quality of the action.

Utilise the wall as support: In Wall Pike, the wall acts as a support, enabling you to retain stability and control at all times. As you maintain appropriate alignment, press your feet firmly against the wall to provide resistance and stability.

Breathing is a crucial component of any workout, especially Wall Pike, so pay attention to it. Exhale as you raise your hips towards the wall and inhale as you drop them into the plank position. Utilise your breathing to strengthen your abdominals and keep your body under control while you exercise.

Increase the challenge gradually: As you become more used to Wall Pike, you may up the degree of difficulty to further test yourself. You may try elevating your hips closer to the wall, or for an even greater challenge, try doing Wall Pike with one leg raised. Always pay attention to your body, and go forward at a rate that is secure for you.

Including Wall Pike in Your Exercise Programme

Here are some pointers on how to add Wall Pike into your exercise programme now that you're aware of its advantages and method:

Warm up properly: Before trying Wall Pike, it's vital to warm up your body. To raise your heart rate and warm up your muscles, start with a few minutes of mild aerobic activity, such brisk walking or cycling. To loosen up your shoulders, hips, and hamstrings, proceed with some dynamic stretches like arm circles and leg swings.

Wall Pike may be a terrific addition to your core exercise programme. Include Wall Pike in your core workout. It may be done as a stand-alone workout or as a component of a circuit. Depending on your fitness level and objectives, aim for 2-3 sets of 8–12 repetitions. Always pay attention to your form and control, and change the challenge level as necessary.

Combine with other exercises: To produce a well-rounded workout, combine Wall Pike with other exercises. It may be used with lower-body movements like squats or lunges, for instance, to produce a full-body workout. As an alternative, you may include it into a whole core training regimen along with other exercises like Russian twists and planks.

As with any workout, it's vital to pay attention to your body. If you feel any pain or discomfort, alter your activity or stop altogether. Before beginning Wall Pike or any new activity, speak with your doctor or a certified fitness expert if you have any pre-existing medical concerns or injuries.

Wall Roll Up for Spinal Mobility and Core Activation

Our general health and well-being are significantly impacted by the spine. It gives our whole body support, balance, and movement. For optimal posture, mobility, and general functioning, maintaining excellent spinal health is crucial. The wall roll up is a useful exercise that may support spinal mobility and core activation. We'll look at the advantages, method, and advice for adding wall rolls to your exercise regimen in this post.

Benefits of Wall Roll Up

Wall Roll Up is a versatile exercise that offers a range of benefits for your body, including:

Spinal Mobility: The Wall Roll Up exercises the spine in a controlled manner, which helps increase spinal mobility. The exercise encourages improved spinal flexibility and range of motion by helping to lengthen and mobilise the vertebrae.

Core Activation: The Wall Roll Up works the deep core muscles, such as the transverse abdominis, obliques, and abdominals. Together, these muscles provide core stability and strength while stabilising the spine.

Improved Posture: Wall Roll Ups may aid posture by strengthening the core muscles that are essential for keeping the spine in the right position. Strong abdominal muscles may support the spine and stop you from hunching over or curving your shoulders.

Muscle Activation: The Wall Roll Up exercise also works the glutes, hamstrings, and hip flexors, which may enhance overall muscle coordination and activation.

minimal Impact: Because the wall roll up has a minimal impact and is easy on the joints, it is appropriate for persons of all ages and fitness levels.

Method for Rolling Up a Wall

The right method for a wall roll-up is shown here:

The first step is to sit on the floor with your back against the wall, your legs out in front of you, and your feet resting on the wall. With your fingers pointed towards your feet, place your hands on the ground behind you.

Keep your legs extended and your feet placed up against the wall as you gently turn over onto your back while engaging your core. Keep your arms flat on the ground behind you.

Breathe in as you raise each vertebra of your spine one at a time. Focus on starting the roll-up from your core, and keep your feet firmly planted on the wall.

Roll yourself up till you are sitting tall and straight. As you get to the peak, let out a breath.

Repeat as many times as necessary while controlling the movement and using appropriate form.

Advice for Executing the Wall Roll Up

Here are some pointers to keep in mind throughout your Wall Roll Up workout to make sure you get the most out of it:

Put your attention on core engagement: Proper core engagement is essential for Wall Roll Up. Avoid utilising momentum or depending on other muscles to do the exercise; instead, make sure your deep core muscles start the action. For optimal efficiency, keep your core engaged throughout the whole action.

Use the wall as a reference: Using the wall as a reference will help you stay in the right alignment for the Wall Roll Up. As you roll up and down, keep your feet firmly planted on the wall for support. By doing so, you can better regulate your movement and avoid putting too much tension on your neck or lower back.

Controlled movement is important while doing the wall roll-up. Focus on keeping a smooth, controlled motion throughout the workout and avoid abrupt movements or swinging. By doing so, you'll be able to activate the target muscles efficiently while lowering your chance of injury.

alter as necessary: To alter the Wall Roll Up, bend your knees and move your feet closer to the wall if you're a novice or have restricted mobility. This might limit the range of motion and make the workout more manageable as you develop your flexibility and strength.

Be mindful of your breathing throughout any workout regimen, including the Wall Roll Up. As you start to roll down, inhale, and as you roll back up, exhale. To strengthen your core and improve the mobility of your body, concentrate on taking slow, deep breaths.

As with any activity, it's crucial to pay attention to your body and to stop if you experience any pain or discomfort. Before beginning the Wall Roll Up or any new activity, speak with a certified fitness expert or healthcare practitioner if you have any pre-existing health issues or injuries.

Adding Wall Roll Ups to Your Workout Routine

You may include the wall roll up to your fitness regimen as a standalone exercise or as a component of a bigger workout. The following suggestions can help you include Wall Roll Ups in your routine:

Warm-up: To get your body ready for activity, start with a simple warm-up. You may engage in some mild cardio for 5 to 10 minutes, such as brisk walking or cycling, and then do some dynamic stretches for your back and abs.

Wall Roll Up: Using good form, do 8–12 repetitions of the exercise while concentrating on engaging your core and moving slowly. If necessary, start with a reduced version and advance progressively as your strength and flexibility improve.

Core exercise: To further engage and improve your core muscles, combine the Wall Roll Up with additional core exercises like planks, Russian twists, or leg raises.

Stretching: To increase flexibility and induce relaxation, end your exercise with some moderate stretches for your spine and core muscles, including the cat-cow posture, child's pose, or the sitting forward fold.

Cool-down: After your exercise, relax your body and mind with a cool-down that includes some static stretches for your main muscle groups and deep breathing.

Always prioritise perfect form, pay attention to your body, and move forward at your own speed. If you're new to exercising or have any worries about your health or fitness level, it's also a good idea to speak with a competent fitness expert.

Wall Mermaid for Side Body Strengthening and Mobility

This unique exercise targets the side body muscles, promoting strength, mobility, and stability.

Benefits of Wall Mermaid

The dynamic Pilates practise known as Wall Mermaid has several health advantages for both the body and the mind. The following are some of the main advantages of include Wall Mermaid in your exercise regimen:

Strengthening of the side of the body: Wall Mermaid concentrates on the obliques, intercostals, and quadratus lumborum. These muscles are essential for maintaining spinal stability, promoting functional movement patterns, and boosting posture.

Core activation: Wall Mermaid works the transverse abdominis, pelvic floor, and multifidus, as do the majority of Pilates movements. Enhancing these muscles may help your everyday activities and overall fitness by enhancing your core stability and control.

Spinal mobility: Wall Mermaid includes lateral spine flexion, which promotes thoracic and lumbar spine mobility. This may help you feel less stiff, be more flexible, and have a wider range of motion for different exercises and activities.

Improved shoulder, chest, and upper back mobility is possible with Wall Mermaid since it also incorporates reaching and stretching motions with the arms. Your posture, respiration, and upper body movement may all improve as a result.

Like other Pilates exercises, Wall Mermaid emphasises the mind-body connection and calls for your presence and awareness of your posture, breathing, and movements. You may improve your body awareness, focus, and relaxation with this.

How to do a wall mermaid

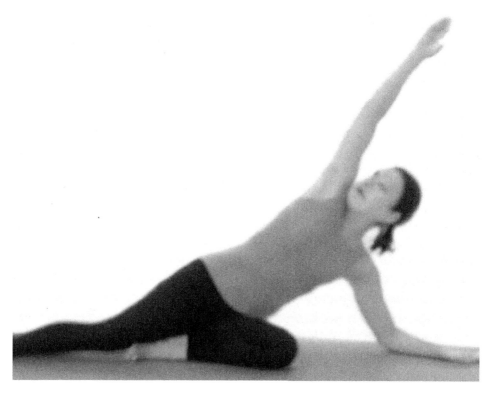

Here is an easy-to-follow guide on how to do Wall Mermaid correctly:

Start by positioning yourself such that your right side is facing a wall and you are approximately a foot away from it. Put your right hand, fingers pointing forward, at shoulder height on the wall. Engage your core and stand tall with your feet hip-width apart.

Inhale to begin, then as you exhale, laterally bend your spine to the right while sliding your right hand along the wall.

Keep your shoulder away from your ear and your arm straight. Keep from sagging into the body's side.

Stretch your left arm up and over your head, forming a long, diagonal line from your fingers to your left foot, while you continue to glide your hand down the wall. Maintain a straight left arm and relaxed shoulders.

Hold the posture with an inhale, then gently exhale to return to the beginning position by tightening your abdominal muscles and raising your hand back up the wall. Keep your motions smooth and in control.

Repeat on the other side: Once you've completed the required number of repetitions on one side, switch to the other side by turning around and doing the exercise the other way.

Modifications for Wall Mermaid

Wall Mermaid may be altered to accommodate various levels of physical fitness and skill. Here are some changes you may want to think about making:

Hand position: If reaching down to the wall is difficult for you, you may start with your hand higher on the wall or complete the exercise using a wall-mounted bar or strap that is positioned higher up.

Range of motion: Depending on your flexibility and degree of comfort, you may change the range of motion. As you grow more at ease and mobile, start with a modest lateral flexion movement and progressively widen the range of motion.

Support: You may rest your other hand gently on the wall or lay it on your hip if you feel unsteady or need more assistance.

Resistance: To increase the difficulty, hold a light dumbbell in the hand that extends above and over, adding extra resistance for the side body muscles.

Tips for Performing Wall Mermaid

Additional pointers for executing Wall Mermaid are provided below:

Pulling your navel towards your spine and keeping your spine in a steady, neutral posture will help you to utilise your deep core muscles throughout the exercise.

Focus on form: Pay close attention to your posture, with your shoulders relaxed, chest up, and neck in a neutral position. Also, pay attention to your alignment.

Breathe rhythmically: Time your breath with your motions, inhaling to get ready and exhaling as you stretch up and over and laterally bend your spine. Refrain from holding your breath or taking short breaths.

Move slowly and deliberately, without hurrying or jerking, and pay attention to the quality of your motions. Throughout the workout, keep your body and mind in the present.

Start with a warm-up: Before beginning any Pilates exercise, it is always a good idea to warm up your body. Spend a few minutes gently stretching and moving your hips, shoulders, and spine.

Adding Wall Mermaid to Your Pilates Exercises

The Pilates exercise known as Wall Mermaid may be a useful addition to your practise since it presents your side body muscles with a special challenge while enhancing mobility, stability, and strength. Incorporate Wall Mermaid into your Pilates workout by using these suggestions:

Exercise that can be done alone: Wall Mermaid may be done alone, adding it to your Pilates regimen as a specific exercise for side body strengthening and mobility.

Exercise for warming up: Wall Mermaid may be used to get your body ready for more difficult Pilates routines. Before beginning additional exercises, do a few repetitions on each side to warm up your spine, shoulders, and hips.

Superset with other exercises: To make your workout more dynamic and difficult, you may combine Wall Mermaid with other Pilates movements. You may, for instance, start with a Wall Mermaid exercise on one side, go to a mat for exercises like Side Plank, Scissor, or Teaser, and then repeat on the other side.

Mix & match: Use your imagination to combine various Pilates moves to build a programme that is unique to your requirements and tastes. For a comprehensive Pilates workout, Wall Mermaid may be paired with other exercises that focus on other muscle regions.

Wall Push-ups for Upper Body Toning and Core Activation

This adaptable exercise is a practical choice for home workouts, vacation, or when you're limited on space since it can be done anyplace with a firm wall. All fitness levels may benefit from wall pushups, which are also readily adapted to meet your strength and capacity.

Benefits of Wall Push-ups

The advantages of wall push-ups for your upper body and core muscles include:

Strength in the upper body: Wall push-ups work the muscles in your chest, shoulders, and triceps, strengthening and toning them.

Your core muscles, including as your abdomen, obliques, and lower back, are activated when you do wall push-ups in order to maintain good form and stability.

Wall push-ups force you to move your shoulders through their entire range of motion, which promotes flexibility and mobility in this joint.

Wall push-ups are an accessible and practical exercise that can be done wherever there is a wall, making them a good choice for home workouts, road trips, and situations where space or equipment is at a premium.

How to Do Push-Ups on the Wall

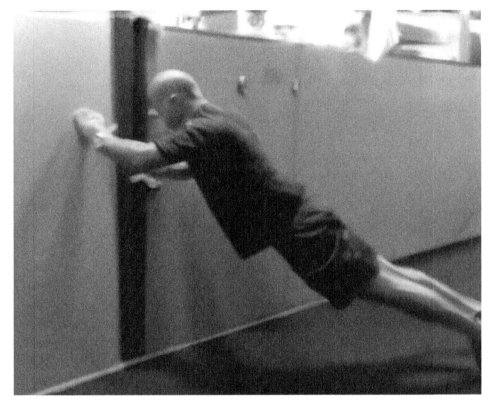

To complete wall push-ups correctly, follow these steps:

Step One

Find a strong wall: Look for a wall that can hold your weight that is level, substantial, and strong. Stand with your feet hip-width apart, facing the wall, and at a distance of approximately an arm's length.

Step Two

Position your hands on the wall so that your fingers are facing upward and they are little broader than shoulder-width apart.

Step Three

Lean forward: To maintain a straight line from your head to your heels, lean your body forward while keeping your feet firmly planted on the ground.

Step Four

Reduce your body's height by bending your elbows and slowly lowering your chest towards the wall while maintaining a straight line with your body. As you lower yourself, try to get your chest or face as near to the wall as possible.

Step Five

Push back up: To go back to the beginning position, push through your hands and straighten your arms while keeping a steady and controlled action.

Step Six

Repeat: Do 10-15 wall push-up reps, or as many as you can with good technique and without strain.

Variations on the wall push-up

To suit your level of fitness and provide diversity to your training programme, you may adapt wall pushups. Here are some alternatives to think about:

Incline push-ups: If wall push-ups are too difficult for you, you may do incline push-ups by putting your hands on a strong bench or step that is inclined. This lowers the exercise's intensity and enables you to gradually increase your strength.

Decline push-ups: You may execute decline push-ups by putting your feet on an elevated platform, such a solid bench or step, and your hands on the wall to make wall push-ups more difficult. Your upper body and core muscles will be under more stress as a result.

Variations in hand placement: You may position your hands differently to stimulate various muscle groups. To work your triceps, for instance, place your hands closer together, while spreading them out to work your chest muscles.

Change the cadence of your wall push-ups to make them more difficult and intense. Try doing moderate, controlled push-ups while concentrating on the eccentric (lowering) phase, or try a plyometric challenge by doing rapid, explosive push-ups.

For more experienced practitioners, you may put yourself to the test by executing one-arm wall push-ups. Push-ups should be done with one hand on the wall while keeping the other behind your back. Your upper body and core need to be stronger and more stable for this variant.

Wall push-ups with a wide stance may be performed by stepping one foot forward and the other back, as opposed to standing with your feet hip-width apart. This broadens your base of support while testing your stability and balance and working additional core muscles.

Close stance wall push-ups: On the other hand, you can also get your toes touching and have a narrower stance when doing push-ups. This works several parts of your chest and triceps while testing your stability and balance.

Including Wall Push-ups in Your Exercise Programme

Push-ups against a wall might be a beneficial addition to any exercise programme. Here are some ideas for successfully incorporating them:

Warm-up: Warming up your muscles before beginning any workout is crucial to lowering the chance of injury. Try some mild exercise for a few minutes, like jumping jacks or brisk walking, and then do some dynamic stretches for your upper body and core.

Start with good form, and keep it up throughout the exercise to make sure you're working the appropriate muscles and lowering your chance of getting hurt. Avoid arching or sagging in your back and keep your body in a straight line while engaging your core.

Increase the intensity gradually. If you're new to wall push-ups or a novice, start with a wall that's closer to you to lessen the difficulty. Increase the distance between you and the wall progressively as your strength and confidence grow to make the workout more difficult.

Observe your body: Pay attention to your body and refrain from exerting too much pressure or sacrificing your form. Rest if you have any pain or discomfort. It's crucial to go forward at your own speed and not push yourself over your present fitness level.

Combine this activity with others: Wall push-ups may be added to other exercises to give your upper body and core a well-rounded workout. For a full-body workout, you may combine them with bodyweight exercises like squats, lunges, or planks.

Like with any fitness programme, persistence is vital to seeing benefits. Wall push-ups should be a part of your weekly exercise regimen at least twice, and as you gain strength, you should progressively raise the quantity or difficulty of repetitions.

Wall Spine Twist for Spinal Mobility and Abdominal Toning

Spinal mobility and core strength are essential for maintaining good posture, preventing back pain, and supporting overall physical health. One effective exercise that can help improve spinal mobility and abdominal tone is the Wall Spine Twist.

How to Perform Wall Spine Twist

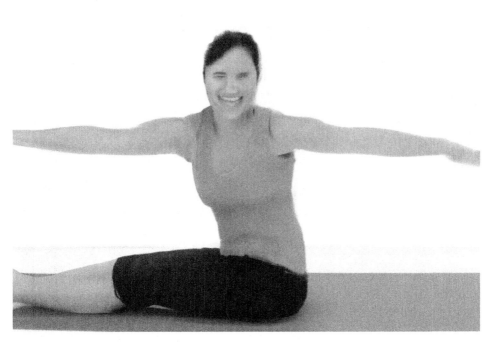

A wall may be used as support for a simple workout called the Wall Spine Twist. How to do it is as follows:

Step One

Locate a free wall area and take a position facing the wall, approximately an arms' length away.

Step Two

Place your palms on the wall with your arms extended straight in front of you at shoulder height.

Step Three

Align your core muscles as you stand tall with your feet hip-width apart.

Step Four

Gently turn your body to the right while maintaining a straight arm position and pushing your hands firmly on the wall. As you twist, let your hips and feet naturally rotate.

Step Five

Hold the twist for a short period of time while feeling your spine and abdominal muscles stretched.

Step Six

Go back to your starting position and then do the left-side twist again.

Step Seven

Complete 10 to 12 repetitions each side, or as many you feel comfortable with.

Variations of Wall Spine Twist

Different fitness levels and objectives may be accommodated by modifying the Wall Spine Twist. You may try these variants, for example:

Sitting Wall Spine Twist: Rather of standing, you may carry out this exercise while sitting, leaning back against the wall and bending your knees. By putting your hands on your thighs and rotating your body to the right and left while keeping perfect form and activating your core, you may improve your balance.

Wall Spine Twist with Extended Arms: To make the twist more difficult, raise your arms in the air. This is a harder variant since it uses more muscles in your shoulders, arms, and upper back.

Bent Knee Wall Spine Twist: You may execute the Wall Spine Twist with your knees slightly bent if you have limited flexibility or range of motion. As a result, your lower back will experience less tension, and those with mobility limitations will find the exercise easier to complete.

Benefits of Wall Spine Twist

The Wall Spine Twist is a flexible workout that has a number of advantages for improving spinal mobility and exercising the abdominal muscles. Among the main advantages are:

Enhanced spinal mobility: The exercise's twisting action aids in mobilising the spine and expanding its range of motion. This may increase general spinal health by reducing stiffness and increasing flexibility.

Muscles of the core, such as the obliques and transverse abdominis, which are in charge of the rotation and stability of the spine, are worked out during the Wall Spine Twist. The abdominal muscles may be toned and strengthened with regular practise of this workout.

Correcting your posture: Back discomfort and other musculoskeletal problems may result from poor posture, which is a frequent condition. By bolstering the muscles that maintain proper posture, such as the core muscles and the muscles around the spine, the Wall Spine Twist may help address postural abnormalities.

Convenience and accessibility: The Wall Spine Twist has the benefit of being performed against a wall, which makes it simple for individuals of all fitness levels. You may do it at home, at the gym, or even while taking a break at work.

Adding Wall Spine Twists to Your Workout Routine

The following advice will help you include the Wall Spine Twist in your exercise routine:

Warm-up: Before beginning the Wall Spine Twist, it's vital to warm up your muscles as you would with any workout. To get your body ready for the workout, you may warm up with a few minutes of mild cardio, like walking or cycling, followed by some dynamic stretches.

Start slowly: When doing the Wall Spine Twist for the first time, move slowly and deliberately. Be careful not to jerk or twist your spine more than it can naturally. As your flexibility and strength grow, gradually up the intensity and range of motion.

Pay attention to form: To maximise the benefits of the Wall Spine Twist and prevent injury, proper form is essential. Maintain a straight back, relaxed shoulders, and active core throughout the exercise. A comfortable range of motion may be found by paying attention to your body and avoiding rounding or arching your back.

Remember to continually and thoroughly inhale and exhale during the workout. As you turn to one side, inhale, and as you come back to the beginning position, exhale. Deep breathing may aid in relaxation and better core muscular engagement.

The Wall Spine Twist may be included into your exercise programme as part of your warm-up, cool-down, or core workout. For a well-rounded workout, it may also be paired with other exercises that concentrate on the upper body and core.

Consult a specialist: Before beginning the Wall Spine Twist or any new workout, it is always essential to speak with a healthcare provider or a competent fitness trainer if you have any pre-existing medical issues or concerns about the health of your spine.

CHAPTER SIX

Nutrition and Lifestyle Strategies for Successful Weight Loss

It might be difficult for many individuals to lose weight. Choosing the best course of action might be difficult with so many alternatives available. But one approach that has become more well-liked recently combines Wall Pilates with dietary and lifestyle recommendations. While attempting to lose weight, wall Pilates may be a useful and pleasurable form of exercise. We'll look at the lifestyle and nutritional approaches that work well with Wall Pilates to assist effective weight reduction, and we'll provide helpful advice on how to apply these approaches to your day-to-day activities.

Why is Nutrition Important for Weight Loss with Wall Pilates?

Nutrition plays a crucial role in weight loss, regardless of the the fitness routine you choose. A well-balanced, nutrient-rich diet will help your weight reduction efforts when paired with Wall Pilates. Here are some important dietary tips to take into account:

Prioritize Whole, unprocessed foods including fruits, vegetables, lean meats, whole grains, and healthy fats should be the mainstay of your diet. In contrast to processed and sugary meals, these foods are fewer in calories and higher in important nutrients, fibre, and antioxidants. They may help you stay satisfied for a longer period of time, reduce cravings, and provide your body the nutrition it needs to operate at its best.

Practise Mindful Eating: Being mindful as you eat means paying attention to your hunger and fullness signs. Eat without being distracted, such as while watching television or using a computer, since this may result in mindless eating and overeating. Spend some time enjoying and savouring your meals, and pay attention to your body's cues to quit when you feel pleasantly full.

Watch Your Portion Sizes: Portion management is crucial for weight reduction, even while eating nutritious meals. Even with wholesome meals, it is simple to overeat. Reduce portion sizes by using smaller dishes and bowls, and minimise mindless eating by avoiding eating directly from a box. Watch your portion sizes while eating high-calorie items like nuts, seeds, avocados, and oils since the calories may add up rapidly.

Keep hydrated Water intake must be enough for weight reduction. A calorie-free beverage that might make you feel satisfied and stop overeating is water. Aim to consume eight to ten glasses of water each day, or more if you exercise. To stay hydrated during the day, you may also include various non-caloric drinks such herbal teas, flavoured water, or sparkling water.

Balance Your Macronutrient consumption: Maintaining a healthy balance between your consumption of carbs, proteins, and fats will help you lose weight. Every meal and snack should have a decent supply of protein, such as tofu or tempeh, or lean meats, fish, eggs, dairy products, or legumes. Instead of refined carbs like white bread, white rice, or sugary meals, choose complex carbohydrates like whole grains, fruits, and vegetables. Include healthy fats in your diet in moderation, such as those found in avocados, nuts, seeds, olive oil, and fatty seafood like salmon and sardines.

Be Wary of Added Sugars: Added sugars might lead to overeating calories and prevent weight reduction. Be aware of added sugars in soda, candy, baked goods, flavoured yoghurt, and sugary cereals, among other meals and drinks. Choose natural sweeteners like fruits or tiny quantities of honey or maple syrup instead of artificial sweeteners.

Plan Your Meals and Snacks: Making better decisions and avoiding impulsive eating are both facilitated by planning your meals and snacks in advance. Based on your dietary requirements and preferred serving sizes, plan your meals and snacks, and make an effort to maintain a regular eating pattern. This may assist in avoiding overeating or making poor food decisions due to excessive hunger.

Limit alcohol intake since it contains a lot of empty calories and might impede weight reduction. When drinking, keep your intake to a minimum and choose for lower-calorie selections. Avoid drinking large quantities of wine or beer or sweet drinks since the calories might pile up.

Seek Professional Advice: It's vital to seek professional guidance from a certified dietitian or nutritionist if you have certain dietary limitations or health concerns. They may provide you personalised advice and suggestions that are catered to your particular requirements and objectives.

How Wall Pilates Lifestyle Changes Can Support Weight Loss

When paired with Wall Pilates, including lifestyle measures in addition to diet might help you lose weight more quickly. Here are some lifestyle suggestions to take into account:

Enhance Your Exercise: Due to the fact that wall Pilates stimulates a variety of muscle groups and may help improve strength, flexibility, and endurance, it has a number of advantages for weight reduction. You may further increase your calorie burn and help weight reduction by combining it with other physical activities, such as cardiovascular workouts like walking, jogging, swimming, or cycling. with addition to Wall Pilates, aim for at least 150 minutes of moderate-intensity aerobic exercise every week to aid with weight reduction and general wellness.

Make Movement a Priority: Make movement a priority in your everyday life in addition to scheduled workouts. Include physical exercise in your daily routine by walking or bicycling to work, using the stairs instead of the lift, parking farther away from your destination, or participating in enjoyable leisure activities. These seemingly little adjustments might add up to a greater daily energy expenditure and aid in weight reduction.

Manage Stress: Stress may hinder attempts at weight reduction by inducing emotional eating or interfering with sleep cycles. Find practical methods for controlling your stress levels, such as deep breathing exercises, yoga, meditation, enough sleep, talking to a therapist or counsellor, or taking part in fun hobbies and activities. You can lessen the chance of emotional eating and assist your weight reduction objectives by controlling your stress.

A healthy lifestyle, including weight reduction, depends on getting enough sleep. The disruption of hunger and fullness signals, an increase in appetite, and changes in metabolism and energy levels may all result from poor sleep or inadequate sleep. To help your attempts to lose weight, aim for 7-9 hours of good sleep each night.

Practise mindfulness: Being aware of your thoughts, feelings, and actions might help you lose weight. Be present when you eat, pay attention to your hunger and fullness signals, refrain from emotional eating, eat slowly and savour each mouthful. Instead of eating out of habit or boredom, pay attention to your body and eat when you are hungry. You may have a healthy connection with food and make better decisions that support your weight reduction objectives by practising mindful eating.

Create a Supportive Environment for Yourself: Your eating patterns and lifestyle decisions are greatly influenced by your surroundings. Create a supportive atmosphere for oneself that promotes healthy habits. Keep wholesome snacks on hand, stock your kitchen with nutritious meals, and keep enticing high-calorie items to a minimum at your home and place of employment. As you embark on your weight reduction journey, surround yourself with encouraging friends, family, or gym partners who can serve as a source of inspiration, accountability, and encouragement.

Engage in Self-Care: Self-care is crucial for achieving weight reduction success. By routinely partaking in things that bring you joy, relaxation, and fulfilment, you may practise self-care. This might involve pastimes, family time away from your hectic schedule, frequent massages, soothing baths, or just having some quiet time to yourself. Setting self-care as a priority may boost your weight reduction goals while reducing stress and enhancing mental health.

Maintain Proper Hydration: Maintaining proper hydration is important for general health and may help you lose weight. Stay hydrated throughout the day by drinking plenty of water, which will make you feel fuller, less hungry, and less inclined to overeat. Avoid sugary drinks like fruit juices and sodas since they might add empty calories to your diet.

Monitor Your Progress: Keeping tabs on your development might inspire you and keep you committed to your weight reduction objectives. Keep track of your dietary consumption, exercise routines, and other lifestyle modifications using a notebook or a mobile app. This may assist you in finding trends, making necessary corrections, and recognising your accomplishments along the route.

Be persistent and patient; sustained effort is necessary for successful weight reduction. It's crucial to have patience with yourself and keep going even if you don't receive results right away. Maintain consistency in your dietary and lifestyle choices, and have faith in the process. Keep in mind that sustained weight reduction is a process, and it's crucial to concentrate on long-term routines rather than temporary remedies.

28 Day Weight Loss Meal Plan

DAY	BREAKFAST	LUNCH	DINNER
1	Greek yogurt with berries and almonds	Grilled chicken salad with mixed greens, vegetables, and balsamic vinaigrette	Baked salmon with roasted vegetables and quinoa
2	Spinach and mushroom omelette with whole grain toast	Lentil and vegetable stir-fry with brown rice	Grilled tofu with steamed broccoli and soba noodles
3	Oatmeal with banana and almond butter	Turkey lettuce wraps with avocado and salsa	Grilled shrimp with roasted Brussels sprouts and sweet potato
4	Greek yogurt with granola and mixed fruit	Quinoa and black bean salad with roasted vegetables	Grilled chicken breast with roasted asparagus and quinoa
5	Veggie-packed smoothie with spinach, banana, Greek yogurt, and almond milk	Grilled vegetable and hummus wrap with whole grain wrap	Baked cod with roasted vegetables and wild rice
6	Whole grain pancakes with berries and Greek yogurt	Chickpea and vegetable curry with brown rice	Grilled turkey burger with lettuce wrap and sweet potato fries
7	Avocado toast with poached eggs and tomato	Lentil and vegetable soup with whole grain bread	Grilled salmon with roasted vegetables and quinoa
8	Cottage cheese with mixed fruit and nuts	Grilled chicken salad with mixed greens, vegetables, and balsamic vinaigrette	Stir-fried tofu with mixed vegetables and brown rice

9	Veggie omelette with mushrooms, peppers, and onions	Quinoa and black bean stuffed bell peppers	Grilled shrimp with roasted vegetables and quinoa
10	Greek yogurt with granola and mixed fruit	Lentil and vegetable stir-fry with brown rice	Baked chicken breast with steamed broccoli and quinoa
11	Overnight chia seed pudding with berries and almond milk	Tofu and vegetable stir-fry with soba noodles	Grilled fish with roasted vegetables and wild rice
12	Whole grain waffles with almond butter and banana	Mediterranean chickpea salad with mixed greens and vinaigrette	Grilled turkey breast with roasted Brussels sprouts and sweet potato
13	Veggie-packed smoothie with spinach, banana, Greek yogurt, and almond milk	Quinoa and roasted vegetable bowl with tahini dressing	Baked cod with roasted vegetables and quinoa
14	Veggie scramble with eggs, peppers, onions, and cheese	Black bean and vegetable chili with whole grain bread	Grilled chicken breast with roasted asparagus and wild rice
15	Greek yogurt with berries and almonds	Lentil and vegetable stir-fry with brown rice	Grilled tofu with steamed broccoli and quinoa
16	Spinach and mushroom omelette with whole grain toast	Chickpea and vegetable curry with brown rice	Grilled fish with roasted vegetables and quinoa
17	Oatmeal with banana and almond butter	Turkey lettuce wraps with avocado and salsa	Baked chicken breast with roasted vegetables and quinoa
18	Greek yogurt with granola and mixed fruit	Veggie and tofu stir-fry with brown rice	Grilled shrimp with roasted vegetables and wild rice
19	Veggie omelette with mushrooms, peppers, and onions	Lentil and vegetable stir-fry with soba noodles	Grilled turkey burger with lettuce wrap and sweet

			potato fries
20	Whole grain pancakes with berries and Greek yogurt	Quinoa and black bean salad with roasted vegetables	Grilled fish with roasted Brussels sprouts and wild rice
21	Avocado toast with poached eggs and tomato	Lentil and vegetable soup with whole grain bread	Grilled chicken breast with roasted vegetables and quinoa
22	Cottage cheese with mixed fruit and nuts	Grilled vegetable and hummus wrap with whole grain wrap	Baked cod with roasted vegetables and wild rice
23	Veggie-packed smoothie with spinach, banana, Greek yogurt, and almond milk	Quinoa and roasted vegetable bowl with tahini dressing	Grilled tofu with steamed broccoli and quinoa
24	Overnight chia seed pudding with berries and almond milk	Chickpea and vegetable stir-fry with brown rice	Grilled fish with roasted vegetables and quinoa
25	Whole grain waffles with almond butter and banana	Mediterranean chickpea salad with mixed greens and vinaigrette	Grilled turkey breast with roasted Brussels sprouts and sweet potato
26	Veggie-packed smoothie with spinach, banana, Greek yogurt, and almond milk	Lentil and vegetable stir-fry with soba noodles	Baked cod with roasted vegetables and quinoa
27	Veggie scramble with eggs, peppers, onions, and cheese	Black bean and vegetable chili with whole grain bread	Grilled chicken breast with roasted asparagus and wild rice
28	Greek yogurt with berries and almonds	Lentil and vegetable stir-fry with brown rice	Grilled tofu with steamed broccoli and quinoa

Printed in Great Britain
by Amazon

21942865R00064